Craving Stability

How Reward Signals, Dopamine Loops, Appetite Pressure, and Reinforcement Patterns Shape Eating Behavior

Nathan Reed

PERENNIAL PUBLISHING

Published by Perennial Publishing

Paperback ISBN: 978-1-971996-63-9
Hardcover ISBN: 978-1-971996-64-6
E-book ISBN: 978-1-971996-65-3

Contents

Craving as a Reinforced Signal

Cravings are among the most familiar and most misinterpreted food-related signals. They are often experienced as urgent, repetitive, emotionally charged, highly specific, and difficult to hold at distance. A craving can narrow attention rapidly. It can interrupt thought, reorganize priority, compress flexibility, and make a particular response feel unusually important within a short period of time. Because the signal feels strong, it is often interpreted morally. The craving becomes evidence of weakness, lack of discipline, emotional instability, poor self-control, addictive tendency, or personal failure.

Intensity becomes identity.

This interpretation is common partly because cravings are felt directly. The signal arrives internally and often carries urgency, specificity, and repetition at the same time. A person may not experience the surrounding structure that amplified the signal. They experience the craving itself. The visible layer becomes the entire explanation. The result is that cravings are frequently interpreted as personal defects rather than as outputs produced by interacting systems of prediction, reinforcement, memory, internal pressure, and learned association.

Craving is not simply hunger, although hunger can intensify it. It is not merely preference, although preference can shape it. It is not simply emotional instability, although emotional strain can amplify it. Craving is better understood as a reinforced signal state shaped by reward expectation, internal pressure, cue exposure, memory, repetition, relief expectation, and system instability.

This distinction matters because interpretation changes what becomes visible.

A craving becomes powerful when prediction, pressure, and repetition begin reinforcing one another.

The point is not that cravings are imaginary, irrational, or meaningless. The intensity is real. The urgency is real. The narrowing effect is real. The repetition can be real. The emotional force can be real. But intensity alone does not explain structure. A strong signal is not automatically moral evidence. A craving may feel overwhelming while still reflecting reinforcement, prediction, relief expectation, stress load, fatigue state, appetite pressure, cue density, or repeated association rather than defective character.

Craving is not proof of weakness. It is evidence that a signal has gained force.

This book approaches craving as a systems phenomenon rather than a moral one. The central question is not whether cravings exist. Human nervous systems are predictive, reward-responsive, associative, and adaptive. Desire, sensory preference, anticipation, and reward sensitivity are ordinary features of regulation and learning. The more useful question is why certain reward signals become amplified, repetitive, emotionally loaded, behaviorally narrowing, and difficult to interpret clearly.

Cravings often become destabilizing when several layers begin converging around the same pathway simultaneously.

Reward expectation is one of those layers. Cravings frequently intensify before eating occurs because the nervous system is already predicting a state change. The anticipated outcome becomes part of the signal itself. A craving may organize around expected pleasure, comfort, stimulation, familiarity, relief, decompression, interruption of boredom, reduction of fatigue, emotional softening, or restoration of perceived stability. The anticipated effect gains salience before the response takes place physically.

The craving is often directed toward what the response is expected to change.

This helps explain why cravings are usually specific rather than broad. Hunger often increases general food relevance. Craving frequently narrows attention toward a particular sensory profile, emotional effect, routine, or context-linked reward expectation. The signal may attach to sweetness, saltiness, crunch, warmth, coldness, creaminess, convenience, familiarity, time of day, emotional atmosphere, or remembered sensory experience. Specificity reveals prediction. The nervous system is not simply asking for intake. It is often anticipating a familiar outcome associated with a particular pathway.

Urgency and specificity therefore become structural clues rather than moral evidence.

The question is not whether the craving is real. The question is what is amplifying it.

Repetition strengthens the same process. When cue, craving, response, reward, relief, and reinforcement repeatedly occur together, the nervous system learns the sequence. Familiar pathways become easier to retrieve because the association has been practiced. A cue repeatedly paired with a rewarding or relieving response gradually becomes more behaviorally relevant. Activation can occur faster because the predictive structure has become more efficient through rehearsal.

Repetition increases retrieval speed.

Over time, the pathway may begin activating before conscious deliberation fully forms. The craving can feel immediate because the nervous system recognizes familiar patterns quickly. Environmental exposure, emotional states, times of day, routines, screens, social settings, smells, locations, fatigue states, and stress conditions may all become linked with anticipated outcomes through repeated pairing.

Cue exposure increases activation opportunities.

Memory deepens the same architecture because the nervous system stores prior associations between reward, relief, emotional tone, context, sensory experience, and expected outcome. A present cue may reactivate an earlier reward pathway before conscious narration catches up. The craving feels immediate partly because memory restores the predictive sequence rapidly. Familiarity gives the signal emotional weight, specificity, and direction.

Memory does not simply recall reward. It restores pathways toward expected reward.

Relief expectation is equally important. Cravings are not reinforced only by pleasure. Reduction of discomfort can become highly reinforcing because nervous systems naturally move toward decreased strain and away from unresolved pressure. A response that repeatedly softens stress, fatigue, boredom, overload, agitation, restriction pressure, emotional strain, or perceived instability may gradually become behaviorally important because it predicts relief.

Relief can strengthen a pathway as strongly as pleasure.

This does not mean the nervous system is malfunctioning. Relief-seeking is not inherently pathological. Under strain, the value of rapid state change increases. The problem is not that relief matters. The problem emerges when repeated reinforcement repeatedly concentrates around the same pathways until the signal becomes increasingly urgent, automatic, repetitive, and behaviorally narrowing.

Internal pressure amplifies the same system further. Appetite pressure, glucose instability, fatigue, sleep debt, stress load, emotional strain, environmental accessibility, and repeated cue exposure can all increase reward salience by raising the value of rapid restoration, familiarity, decompression, convenience, or low-friction relief. A signal that might remain manageable under lower-pressure conditions can become highly persuasive when several amplification systems converge simultaneously.

Stress increases relief value. Fatigue increases the value of ease. Glucose instability increases urgency around rapid restoration. Sleep debt narrows emotional margin and increases reward sensitivity. Appetite pressure increases the force of reward relevance. Environmental availability increases cue contact and lowers response friction. Memory increases retrieval efficiency. Repetition increases automaticity.

The pathway gains force because amplification layers begin reinforcing one another.

When craving is interpreted morally, these surrounding layers disappear from view. The signal becomes reduced to character. The person appears to be the problem instead of the amplification structure surrounding the signal. But cravings are often more understandable when interpreted as outputs produced by interacting systems rather than as evidence of personal defect.

Interpretation changes clarity.

This shift does not require denying agency, minimizing responsibility, or treating cravings as meaningless reflexes. The nervous system remains adaptive, predictive, and behaviorally responsive throughout ordinary life. The point is structural accuracy. Cravings become easier to interpret when viewed as reinforced signals shaped by prediction, memory, repetition, internal pressure, and environmental exposure rather than as isolated evidence of weakness.

Craving stability emerges from this same frame.

Craving stability does not mean the elimination of desire, reward sensitivity, pleasure, appetite, sensory interest, or wanting. Human nervous systems remain reward-responsive under stable conditions. Desire continues to exist because reward remains part of learning, adaptation, pleasure, regulation, and ordinary behavior. Stability is not emotional neutrality around food. It is not permanent absence of craving. It is not total freedom from reward signals.

Craving stability means reduced amplification.

The signal becomes less urgent, less repetitive, less behaviorally narrowing, and less emotionally dominant because fewer systems repeatedly intensify the same pathway at the same time. Desire may remain present while urgency decreases. Reward may remain meaningful while repetition loses force. Memory may remain recognizable while salience softens. Familiarity may persist while automaticity weakens.

The opposite of craving instability is not control. It is lower amplification.

Seen through this lens, cravings become more readable. Specificity reveals prediction. Urgency reveals amplification. Repetition reveals reinforcement density. Relief-seeking reveals internal pressure. Cue activation reveals learned association. Emotional force reveals convergence across systems rather than proof of personal weakness.

The signal becomes understandable when the surrounding structure becomes visible.

Cravings often feel confusing because the amplification systems shaping them remain hidden beneath the experience itself. But when craving is interpreted as a reinforced signal state shaped by reward expectation, memory, repetition, cue exposure, internal pressure, and relief prediction, the signal begins to separate from morality. The craving no longer has to function as evidence about identity, discipline, or worth. It becomes information about reinforcement, salience, pressure, prediction, and system coordination.

Craving becomes less morally confusing when the amplification systems surrounding it can finally be seen clearly.

Signal Amplification Mechanism

Cravings are often interpreted as evidence. Evidence of weak discipline. Evidence of emotional instability. Evidence of poor control, excessive desire, lack of restraint, or personal failure. The experience itself can feel persuasive enough to support those conclusions. A craving may arrive with urgency, repetition, specificity, and psychological weight. It may interrupt attention, narrow focus, increase tension, and return repeatedly even when ignored. Because the signal feels strong, the interpretation often becomes moral. The intensity is treated as proof that something is wrong with the person experiencing it.

This interpretation is common partly because cravings feel unusually personal. They appear inside conscious experience. They create mental pull. They may seem emotionally loaded, irrational, embarrassing, excessive, or disproportionate. Unlike many physiological signals that operate quietly in the background, cravings often enter awareness directly. They feel active rather than passive. They can seem to argue, insist, pressure, or demand. The subjective intensity of the experience encourages identity-based interpretation. The signal becomes attached to character.

This book begins from a different frame.

A craving is better understood as an amplified signal state.

This does not reduce the intensity of the experience. Cravings can be powerful. They can feel behaviorally narrowing and difficult to ignore. They can become repetitive, intrusive, emotionally charged, and highly specific. The point is not that cravings are weak signals being exaggerated unnecessarily by the person experiencing them. The point is that strong signals are not automatically moral evidence. Intensity does not explain itself. A signal can become intensified for structural reasons.

The body and brain continuously produce signals related to energy availability, anticipated reward, environmental relevance, prior reinforcement, emotional salience, stress load, recovery state, and behavioral prediction. Most of these signals remain mild, diffuse, flexible, or temporary. Some remain informational without becoming urgent. Others become amplified. The difference matters.

An ordinary desire may remain broad and negotiable. A person may notice interest in food, comfort, stimulation, novelty, or pleasure without experiencing pressure. The signal exists, but it does not dominate attention. It remains flexible enough to move in and out of awareness without creating urgency. It may carry preference without insistence.

An intensified craving behaves differently.

The signal becomes more specific. More repetitive. More urgent. Attention begins to narrow around a particular anticipated outcome. The craving no longer merely suggests that something could be rewarding or useful. It begins to imply that relief, regulation, comfort, energy, familiarity, or satisfaction are closely tied to a specific response. The signal gains behavioral pull.

This shift from ordinary signal to amplified craving is the foundation of the Signal Amplification Mechanism.

The Signal Amplification Mechanism describes the process by which an ordinary desire, cue, appetite signal, memory, or reward expectation becomes intensified when internal pressure and contextual reinforcement converge. The signal becomes stronger not because the individual has suddenly become morally weaker, but because amplification conditions have increased the urgency, salience, and predicted value of the anticipated response.

Signals do not emerge in isolation. They emerge within system state.

A craving that appears suddenly often has a longer structural background than the moment itself suggests. Internal conditions may already be increasing sensitivity before conscious awareness recognizes the craving. Fatigue may already be narrowing tolerance. Stress load may already be increasing pressure for relief. Glucose variability may already be increasing instability in perceived energy availability. Appetite pressure may already be elevated. Sleep debt may already be reducing regulatory flexibility. Emotional strain may already be increasing the perceived value of comfort, familiarity, or distraction. The craving may appear conscious only after multiple amplification layers are already active.

At the same time, contextual conditions shape how signals are interpreted and intensified. Environment matters because the nervous system does not evaluate signals independently from surroundings. A cue associated with prior reward can increase salience before conscious analysis occurs. Smell, location, time of day, screen exposure, routine, social setting, memory, availability, and repeated associations can increase the probability that certain signals become amplified. The context helps determine which signals become foregrounded and which remain quiet.

The resulting craving may feel immediate, but amplification often begins before the moment feels visible.

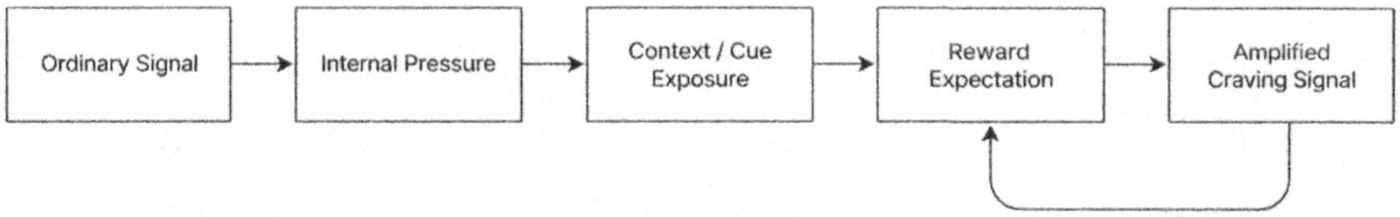

[Figure 1: Signal Amplification Pathway]

The pathway matters because cravings are commonly interpreted only at their endpoint. The amplified signal becomes visible, but the amplification process remains hidden. The person experiences the urgency but not necessarily the layered conditions that increased the urgency. This creates the illusion that cravings emerge spontaneously from character rather than from interacting pressures.

The misunderstanding becomes stronger because amplified signals often feel unusually specific. Hunger may remain broad. Cravings often narrow. The signal may become attached to a particular food, experience, sensory pattern, or anticipated emotional outcome. The narrowing itself contributes to the feeling of urgency. The system no longer merely registers possible usefulness. It begins predicting a specific form of resolution.

This specificity is important because amplified signals frequently carry expected outcomes in addition to anticipated pleasure. A craving is not always simply a pursuit of enjoyment. The anticipated outcome may involve regulation, familiarity, relief from cognitive fatigue, interruption of emotional discomfort, stimulation during low energy, reduction of internal tension, or temporary escape from pressure. The expected effect can become part of the signal itself.

Reward expectation increases amplification because anticipation changes system priority before any behavior occurs.

The nervous system continuously predicts outcomes. When a particular response becomes associated with relief, comfort, pleasure, stimulation, or emotional softening, the anticipated outcome itself can increase signal intensity. The craving becomes partially future-oriented. The system begins moving toward a predicted state improvement before the improvement actually occurs.

This matters because the experience of craving is often interpreted too narrowly as desire for the object itself. In many cases, the signal includes anticipated change in internal state. The expected outcome may involve quieting mental strain, interrupting boredom, softening emotional discomfort, increasing alertness, creating familiarity, reducing heaviness, or restoring perceived reward availability. The anticipated effect becomes attached to the cue.

As anticipation strengthens, the signal can become increasingly behaviorally persuasive. Attention narrows further. Competing priorities become quieter. The anticipated response begins to feel disproportionately important relative to the broader environment. Again, this does not mean the person has suddenly become irrational or morally compromised. It means the signal has become amplified.

Internal pressure contributes significantly to amplification conditions.

Pressure does not refer only to obvious emotional distress. The body continuously manages competing demands related to energy regulation, recovery, attention, emotional processing, environmental adaptation, and physiological stability. Signals change under these conditions. A fatigued system does not interpret reward identically to a well-rested system. A system under chronic stress load does not evaluate comfort, stimulation, or relief identically to a system operating with high recovery capacity.

Hunger can increase signal intensity, but cravings cannot be reduced to hunger alone. Fatigue may increase the pull toward fast reward, stimulation, or familiarity. Glucose variability may increase perceived urgency surrounding quick availability. Sleep debt may reduce regulatory flexibility while increasing sensitivity to reward-associated cues. Emotional strain may increase the anticipated value of distraction, comfort, or interruption. Restriction pressure may increase cognitive salience around previously constrained responses. Under-recovery may reduce resilience against amplification conditions that would otherwise remain mild.

These layers do not operate independently. They interact.

A fatigued person under stress, operating on low recovery, exposed to repeated reward cues, and anticipating relief may experience a dramatically different signal intensity than the same person under lower pressure conditions. The amplified craving reflects the combined state rather than a single variable.

This interaction helps explain why cravings can fluctuate across time even when the external cue appears similar. A food, environment, memory, or routine that feels insignificant one day may feel highly compelling another day. The difference is not necessarily inconsistency of character. The amplification conditions changed.

Context further shapes amplification by increasing cue salience.

Human behavior does not occur in neutral sensory space. Repeated associations matter because the nervous system learns patterns of predicted relevance. Time of day can become associated with anticipated reward. Certain environments can increase expectation automatically. Visual exposure, smells, social routines, screens, entertainment patterns, and repeated pairings between specific experiences and relief can all increase amplification probability.

The cue itself may eventually trigger anticipation before conscious intention appears. This does not require dramatic conditioning language to become meaningful. Repetition naturally changes signal accessibility. A repeatedly reinforced pathway becomes easier to activate later because the anticipated outcome becomes increasingly familiar and cognitively available.

Importantly, amplification does not mean inevitability. The existence of a strong signal does not erase agency. But this book is not primarily concerned with proving that people can resist cravings. The more important issue is interpretation. When amplification is misunderstood as personal defect, the signal becomes psychologically distorted.

Judgment changes interpretation quality.

Once cravings become moralized, system information collapses into identity language. The question shifts away from structural conditions and toward self-condemnation. Instead of asking what pressures may be increasing amplification, the interpretation becomes centered around perceived weakness, failure, lack of discipline, or inability to control oneself.

This shift matters because moral interpretation often obscures the actual structure of the signal.

A person may recognize the craving itself while missing the surrounding conditions entirely. Fatigue disappears from interpretation. Recovery debt disappears. Stress load disappears. Cue exposure disappears. Repetition disappears. Anticipated relief disappears. The amplified signal is stripped from context and interpreted as personality.

The result is reduced clarity.

The craving becomes harder to understand because the analysis no longer examines amplification conditions. Judgment compresses a multi-layered signal into a moral conclusion. The signal may even become more psychologically charged because shame itself can increase internal strain, emotional pressure, and cognitive fixation surrounding the craving experience.

This does not mean judgment creates all cravings. It means judgment can intensify confusion surrounding them.

The distinction matters because understanding amplification is different from approving every impulse. Interpreting cravings as signals does not require romanticizing them, obeying them automatically, or pretending they are harmless. The purpose of interpretation is not permission. The purpose is clarity.

A craving can be real without being authoritative.

The signal may carry information without requiring fear or moral collapse. It may indicate accumulated pressure, narrowed recovery margin, elevated reward sensitivity, repeated reinforcement, or contextual amplification. None of these explanations require the person to become the signal itself.

The seriousness of cravings is often misunderstood because people assume only two interpretations are available. Either cravings are meaningless and should be ignored entirely, or cravings are evidence of deep personal weakness. Both interpretations reduce clarity.

A signal can matter structurally without becoming moral evidence.

This distinction becomes especially important because amplified cravings often coexist with conflict. A person may simultaneously experience strong behavioral pull and strong resistance. The resulting tension is commonly interpreted as proof of dysfunction. But conflicting signals are not unusual within complex systems. Different priorities can become active simultaneously. Long-term goals, short-term regulation, anticipated reward, social identity, fatigue state, emotional strain, and environmental cues may all influence interpretation at once.

The experience can therefore feel internally divided without requiring a moral explanation.

Cravings also become easier to misread because amplification tends to narrow temporal perspective. Immediate anticipated relief can temporarily overshadow broader context. The system prioritizes predicted short-term resolution. This narrowing effect is part of amplification itself. The signal becomes louder partly because competing information becomes quieter.

Again, this does not mean the person loses all capacity for reflection. It means amplification changes relative salience.

The nervous system continuously prioritizes information according to perceived relevance, anticipated reward, predicted relief, and survival-related significance. Under conditions of elevated pressure, reward-associated signals may temporarily rise in priority. The resulting craving feels urgent because the system is allocating attention accordingly.

Repetition further stabilizes amplification pathways over time.

When a particular signal is repeatedly associated with a rewarding or relieving response, future activation may occur more easily. The system increasingly predicts the anticipated outcome. Familiar pathways become cognitively accessible with less prompting. Certain cues begin carrying predictive weight before conscious reasoning fully engages.

This process does not need to be dramatized into deterministic language. Human behavior remains variable and context-dependent. But repetition changes probability. Signals repeatedly paired with reinforcement tend to become more available later. Anticipation becomes easier to trigger. Context becomes more behaviorally meaningful. The pathway becomes more familiar.

The important point for this chapter is not to fully map reinforcement dynamics yet. The important point is to establish that cravings intensify structurally. They are shaped by interaction between internal pressure, contextual exposure, anticipated reward, repetition, and interpretation.

The signal itself is not the whole story.

Cravings become easier to understand once they are repositioned from morality into mechanism. The urgency may still exist. The repetition may still exist. The specificity may still exist. But the meaning changes. The signal is no longer treated as proof of personal failure. It becomes information about amplification conditions operating within the system.

This reframing matters because interpretation changes what becomes visible.

When cravings are interpreted morally, the person mainly sees identity threat. When cravings are interpreted structurally, pressure patterns become easier to recognize. The focus shifts from condemnation toward observation. Internal state, context, repetition, reward expectation, recovery strain, and amplification conditions become conceptually available again.

The craving itself may still feel powerful. But power alone does not define meaning.

A loud signal is not necessarily a truthful signal about character. It may instead reflect accumulated pressure, reinforced expectation, narrowed recovery capacity, repeated association, heightened salience, or intensified predicted reward value. The amplified state reflects system conditions interacting across time.

Cravings therefore do not need to be treated as commands, feared as moral failures, or dismissed as meaningless noise. They can be interpreted.

That interpretation begins by recognizing amplification.

Once craving is understood as an amplified signal state rather than evidence of broken character, the experience becomes structurally readable. The relevant questions change. Instead of asking why a person lacks discipline, attention can shift toward understanding how hunger, reward expectation, memory, repetition, cue exposure, stress load, fatigue, recovery state, and contextual reinforcement interact to increase signal intensity.

The craving remains real. The urgency remains real. The pull remains real. But the interpretation becomes more precise.

The signal is carrying information about pressure within the system.

Hunger-Craving Separation Mechanism

Hunger and craving are often treated as the same experience because both can involve food, attention, urgency, bodily pressure, and mental repetition. Each can make food more noticeable. Each can narrow attention around intake. Each can create the sense that something is needed, missing, unfinished, or unresolved. Because they often appear near each other, they are easily collapsed into one category. The person feels pressure around food, and the pressure is interpreted as hunger. Or the person feels a specific pull toward something rewarding, and that pull is treated as the same thing as appetite. The overlap is real, but overlap does not mean sameness.

Hunger and craving can appear together, influence each other, and blend into one felt experience, but they do not carry identical information. Hunger generally points toward broad energy relevance. It signals that fuel, intake, availability, or depletion may matter to the system. Craving often points toward reward specificity. It signals that a particular remembered, expected, cued, or reinforced outcome has become salient. Hunger may open the field toward food in general. Craving often narrows the field toward a specific food, sensory profile, ritual, context, or expected form of relief.

The difference is not absolute. Hunger is not always vague, and craving is not always detached from energy need. A person can be genuinely hungry and also crave something specific. A craving can become stronger when hunger is present. Hunger can give the signal pressure, while craving gives the signal direction. But the distinction remains important because the two signals are organized differently. One is usually broader. The other is usually more targeted. One often relates to energy need. The other often relates to reward expectation, memory, cue association, relief prediction, or reinforced context.

This is the function of the Hunger-Craving Separation Mechanism. The Hunger-Craving Separation Mechanism is the process of distinguishing broad energy-seeking signals from specific reward-seeking signals so craving can be interpreted as a reinforced signal state rather than being confused with ordinary hunger or moral failure. The mechanism does not divide human experience into clean categories. It creates interpretive clarity inside a mixed signal environment.

Hunger, in its broadest form, is an energy signal. It indicates that intake may be relevant. It may appear as emptiness, low availability, declining tolerance, increased food awareness, reduced patience, or a general openness toward eating. It does not always announce itself dramatically. It may rise gradually. It may become more noticeable when intake has been delayed, when energy demand has increased, when prior intake was insufficient, or when recovery conditions are strained. Its structure is often wide rather than narrow. Food in general becomes relevant.

Craving has a different signature. It often has a target. It may attach to a specific taste, texture, temperature, brand, setting, time of day, routine, or remembered effect. It may not simply communicate that food would be useful. It may communicate that this particular thing, in this particular form, would produce a particular expected state. That expected state may be pleasure, comfort, stimulation, familiarity, relief, regulation, distraction, or emotional softening. The craving becomes specific because the signal is not only about intake. It is also about anticipated reward.

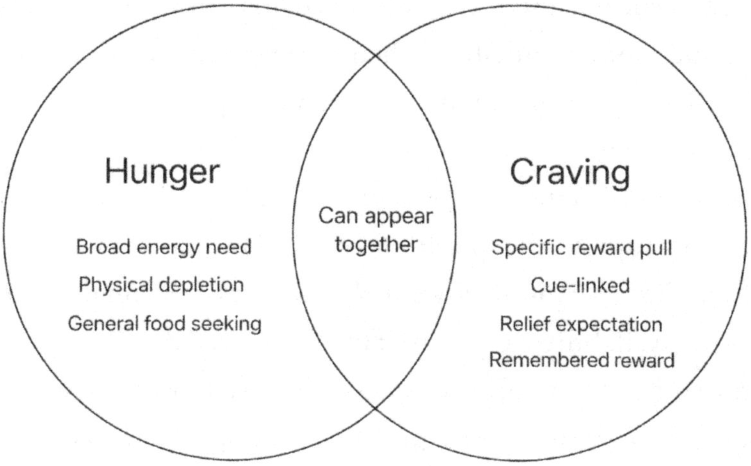

[Figure 2: Hunger vs Craving Signal Map]

The distinction becomes clearer when hunger is understood as broad and craving as shaped by specificity. Hunger may make many foods acceptable. Craving often makes one kind of food feel unusually relevant. Hunger may create general food-seeking. Craving may create a narrowed reward image. Hunger may be satisfied by adequacy. Craving may remain attached to a predicted sensory or emotional outcome. Hunger asks for availability. Craving often asks for a remembered pattern.

This does not make craving false. A craving is not unreal because it is specific. Specificity is part of the signal's structure. The mistake is interpreting specificity as proof of weakness or interpreting hunger as the only legitimate form of food-related pressure. A craving can be real without being the same as hunger. It can carry information without being reducible to energy need.

Hunger can intensify craving because the system under energy pressure becomes more sensitive to reward. When availability feels low, when appetite pressure has accumulated, or when the interval since intake has stretched beyond the system's current tolerance, reward signals may gain force. A cue that might have remained mild under stable conditions can become more compelling when hunger is present. The body is already oriented toward intake, so a reward-specific signal has more pressure behind it.

In this blended state, hunger supplies the broad biological pressure while craving supplies the specific direction. The person may not simply want food. The person may want the food most strongly associated with rapid availability, pleasure, familiarity, relief, or prior reward. The craving feels more urgent because the system is not starting from neutrality. It is already under pressure. The specific reward signal is being amplified by a broader energy signal.

This is one reason cravings can become stronger during long gaps, unstable intake patterns, inadequate satiety, or periods of high demand. The craving may appear to be about one food, but its force may be partly carried by hunger. The specific target is not the whole signal. Beneath it may be a broader state of appetite pressure or perceived depletion. The craving has a direction, but hunger may be providing momentum.

At the same time, cravings can appear without true hunger. This is essential to the separation. A craving may be triggered by context, memory, routine, emotional pressure, stress, fatigue, sleep debt, screen exposure, availability, smell, social setting, or repeated association even when broad energy need is not especially high. The system may not be seeking fuel in a general sense. It may be responding to a cue-linked expectation.

A familiar evening environment may activate a craving because the setting has been repeatedly paired with a certain reward. A stressful transition may activate a craving because the system anticipates relief. Fatigue may increase the appeal of stimulation or convenience. A memory may bring back the expected comfort of a specific sensory experience. A social context may increase salience around a repeated pattern. In these cases, the craving is not imaginary, but it is not identical to hunger. It is a specific reward signal activated by conditions other than energy need.

This is why conflating hunger and craving reduces clarity. If every craving is called hunger, the reward-specific structure disappears from view. Cue association, memory, relief expectation, habit, stress load, and reinforced context remain hidden. The person may keep interpreting the signal as simple energy need even when the craving is being carried by anticipation, familiarity, or environmental repetition.

The opposite error also matters. If hunger is always dismissed as craving, genuine energy need may be overlooked. A person may interpret broad depletion as mere reward-seeking. General food-seeking may be mislabeled as lack of control. The system may be communicating ordinary need, but the interpretation becomes suspicious. Hunger becomes distrusted because craving has been moralized. This too reduces clarity.

The purpose of separating hunger from craving is not self-policing. It is not a rule system. It is not a method for deciding which signals are acceptable. It is a way of reading structure. Hunger and craving can both be real. They can coexist without one invalidating the other. The presence of craving does not make hunger false. The presence of hunger does not erase reward specificity. Separation simply allows each layer to be seen more accurately.

Blended signals are common because the body does not organize experience into isolated categories. A person can be hungry, fatigued, stressed, exposed to cues, remembering prior reward, anticipating relief, and operating inside a familiar routine all at once. The resulting signal may feel like one unified pressure, but it may contain multiple components. Hunger may be present as general intake relevance. Craving may be present as specificity. Stress may add urgency. Fatigue may reduce tolerance. Memory may provide the target. Context may trigger the expectation.

In a blended signal, the craving often feels stronger than hunger alone because it is more organized around a predicted outcome. Hunger may create openness. Craving creates direction. The system does not merely register that food could help. It predicts that a particular response will produce a particular effect. That prediction concentrates attention. The more concentrated the signal becomes, the more it may feel like necessity.

This narrowing can be mistaken for proof. The person may assume that because the signal is specific, the specific thing must be needed. But specificity does not always mean biological necessity. It often means learned relevance, expected reward, or reinforced association. The system is predicting value. Prediction is not the same as requirement.

Hunger, by contrast, may be less tied to a single object. It may not care as much about a particular texture, flavor, brand, or ritual. It may respond to adequacy rather than specificity. This is not always perfectly true, especially when hunger becomes intense, but it remains a useful distinction. Hunger widens the relevance of food. Craving narrows relevance around a particular expected reward.

The distinction also helps explain why a craving can persist after sufficient intake. If the craving was mainly reward-specific, energy intake alone may not fully resolve the expected reward signal. The body may no longer be broadly hungry, but the anticipated sensory, emotional, or contextual outcome may remain active. This does not make the craving mysterious. It means the signal was not only about fuel.

Conversely, a craving may fade when hunger is addressed because the reward-specific signal was being amplified by appetite pressure. Once broad energy pressure decreases, the craving may lose force. In that case, hunger was not the same as craving, but it was contributing to the craving's intensity. The relationship is interactive rather than binary.

The Hunger-Craving Separation Mechanism therefore protects against oversimplification. It prevents hunger from being reduced to craving and craving from being reduced to hunger. It also prevents craving from being reduced to morality. Once the signal is separated structurally, the question becomes less accusatory and more precise. What kind of signal is active? Is the pressure broad or specific? Is the system communicating general energy relevance, or is it predicting reward, relief, familiarity, or context-linked satisfaction?

These questions are interpretive, not prescriptive. They do not instruct a response. They clarify the signal.

This distinction is especially important in a culture that often gives hunger and craving different moral status. Hunger may be treated as legitimate while craving is treated as indulgent, suspicious, or evidence of poor control. That hierarchy distorts interpretation. Craving is not morally inferior to hunger. It is simply structured differently. Hunger may relate more directly to energy need. Craving may relate more directly to reward expectation and reinforcement. Both are signals. Neither is a verdict.

When craving is moralized, the person may try to prove that the craving is really hunger in order to make the signal acceptable. Or the person may deny hunger because the presence of craving makes the whole experience feel suspect. Both responses blur the system. The signal becomes entangled with identity rather than interpreted through structure.

A more stable interpretation does not require suspicion. It requires separation.

Hunger tells part of the story. Craving tells another part. Appetite pressure may increase the volume. Reward expectation may define the target. Memory may supply familiarity. Cue association may bring the signal forward. Stress and fatigue may increase urgency. Repetition may make the pathway easier to activate. Context may determine why the signal appears in one setting and not another.

Seen this way, a craving is not an enemy of hunger. Hunger is not a defense against craving. They are different signal forms that can overlap inside the same experience. Their interaction can be strong, but their meanings are not identical.

The separation becomes most useful when the craving feels urgent. Urgency tends to collapse interpretation. The signal appears strong, and strength is mistaken for simplicity. But an urgent food-related signal may contain broad hunger, reward specificity, relief expectation, memory, routine, stress load, and contextual reinforcement at the same time. Its intensity does not prove that it has only one cause. It often means multiple layers are converging.

The clearer the separation, the easier it becomes to understand amplification. Hunger may amplify craving. Craving may appear without hunger. Hunger and craving may blend. Mislabeling either one reduces clarity. None of these distinctions require shame, control language, or rigid rules. They require a more accurate reading of what the system is communicating.

Hunger and craving are not enemies. They are not moral categories. They are signals with different structures. Hunger generally points toward broad energy relevance. Craving often points toward specific reward expectation, remembered relief, cue association, or reinforced context. When they overlap, the signal may become more intense. When they separate, the difference becomes visible.

A craving does not need to be treated as fake hunger. Hunger does not need to be dismissed because craving is present. Each signal can be real. Each can carry information. The value of separation is that craving becomes more readable as an amplified, reinforced signal rather than a personal defect or a disguised version of every food-related need.

Once hunger and craving are separated without turning them against each other, craving pressure becomes easier to understand. Its intensity can be traced not only to energy need, but to reward specificity, relief expectation, memory, cue exposure, internal state, and repeated context. The signal remains serious, but it becomes less morally loaded. It becomes information about how broad appetite pressure and specific reward pull interact within the system.

Specificity Mechanism

One of the clearest indications that craving is structurally different from ordinary hunger is specificity. Hunger often broadens the relevance of food. A hungry system may become generally interested in intake, availability, energy restoration, or relief from depletion. Craving behaves differently. Craving frequently narrows attention toward a particular target. The signal becomes more selective. It may organize itself around a specific food, texture, flavor, temperature, timing pattern, emotional state, environment, ritual, or remembered effect. The narrowing itself is meaningful.

A person experiencing broad hunger may feel open toward many forms of intake. A person experiencing craving often feels pulled toward something more precise. Not simply sweetness, but a certain type of sweetness. Not simply warmth, but a familiar warm food associated with comfort or decompression. Not simply food in general, but a particular combination of texture, convenience, sensory profile, timing, and expected effect. The specificity of the signal reveals that craving is not only about fuel availability. It is shaped by prediction, association, memory, reinforcement, and learned context.

This narrowing process is the Specificity Mechanism.

The Specificity Mechanism describes the process by which craving organizes itself around a particular sensory profile, timing pattern, routine, context, memory, or expected effect because the system has learned to associate that target with reward, relief, stimulation, familiarity, or regulation. The signal becomes more directed because the anticipated outcome becomes more organized. The craving no longer simply communicates that something would be rewarding. It begins predicting that this specific thing, in this specific form, under these specific conditions, is associated with a meaningful outcome.

Specificity matters because it reveals structure. If cravings were only expressions of broad biological need, they would tend to remain less selective. But cravings often arrive with detailed preference. The system may not simply seek intake. It may seek crunch, warmth, coldness, saltiness, sweetness, creaminess, softness, richness, speed, convenience, familiarity, stimulation, or completion of a ritual pattern. The signal gains precision because the anticipated reward has become associated with particular sensory and contextual features.

This does not make those features inherently problematic. Texture is not morally dangerous. Sweetness is not evidence of failure. Salt, fat, warmth, crunch, coldness, creaminess, speed of access, convenience, and sensory intensity are simply characteristics that the nervous system can associate with reward, familiarity, relief, or expected regulation. The point is not that certain foods are "bad" because they are craved. The point is that specificity itself provides information about how the system learns prediction.

A craving for something warm after emotional strain may not only concern temperature. Warmth may be associated with comfort, slowing down, familiarity, or reduction of tension. A craving for something crunchy during stress may not only concern texture. The sensory intensity and interruption pattern may carry expected stimulation or relief. A craving for something rapidly accessible may not only concern convenience. Speed may matter because the anticipated state change feels urgent. The specificity reveals the predicted effect.

This is why cravings often feel unusually convincing. The signal is not broad and abstract. It is organized around remembered outcomes.

The more tightly the expected effect becomes associated with a particular sensory profile, the more focused the craving may become.

A craving may therefore carry multiple layers simultaneously. The sensory target may include flavor, texture, temperature, timing, ritual, emotional association, and environmental familiarity all at once. The person may consciously notice only the food itself while the system is also predicting decompression, stimulation, comfort, familiarity, interruption of fatigue, reduction of boredom, or completion of a routine. The specificity concentrates the signal.

The narrowing process also explains why cravings often feel less interchangeable than hunger. A broadly hungry person may accept many forms of intake. A craving may remain unsatisfied even after sufficient food if the expected sensory or contextual pattern was not addressed. This does not mean the specific target was biologically necessary. It means the anticipated reward prediction remained active.

Specificity is therefore not proof of need. It is evidence of organized expectation.

The distinction matters because specificity is frequently misinterpreted. A highly specific craving can feel so persuasive that the specific object begins to seem uniquely required. But prediction and necessity are not identical. The nervous system may predict that a certain target is associated with reward, comfort, familiarity, or relief without that target representing an essential biological requirement. The specificity reflects learned association more than objective necessity.

At the same time, specificity should not be dismissed as meaningless. The signal becomes organized for a reason. The system has learned that certain combinations of sensory experience, timing, emotional context, and environmental exposure tend to produce particular outcomes. The craving carries the memory of those associations forward into anticipation.

This process develops gradually across repeated exposure and repeated context. A sensory pattern repeatedly paired with relief, pleasure, stimulation, comfort, or regulation becomes increasingly recognizable. Over time, the nervous system begins predicting the expected effect before the response occurs. The craving therefore arrives not only as desire, but as anticipation.

The anticipatory nature of craving helps explain why specificity can become remarkably detailed. A person may crave not simply sweetness, but a specific type of sweetness associated with a particular emotional or contextual memory. The craving may become attached to a certain texture, brand, preparation style, location, timing pattern, or social environment because the predicted reward was repeatedly experienced in those conditions. The specificity becomes sharper because the prediction becomes more refined.

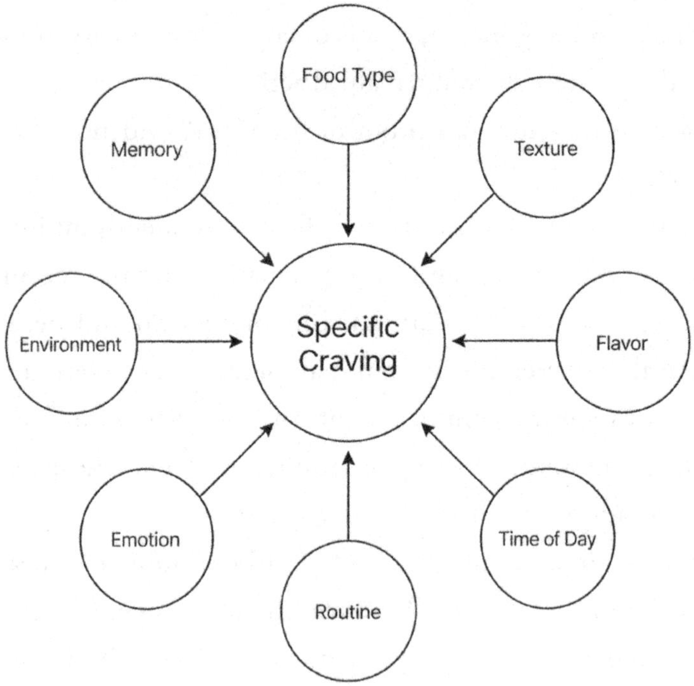

[Figure 3: Craving Specificity Web]

Timing plays a significant role in specificity because repeated rhythms become associated with expected outcomes. A craving that appears at a certain time of day is not necessarily caused by the clock itself. More often, the time represents an established context. Evening may become associated with decompression. The end of work may become associated with release from cognitive demand. Screen time may become associated with stimulation, comfort, or disengagement from effort. Driving routes, weekend transitions, social gatherings, and post-meal routines may all develop predictive associations over time.

The repetition matters because the nervous system learns continuity between cue and outcome. If a particular sensory experience repeatedly appears during a predictable transition state, anticipation may begin activating before conscious intention fully forms. The signal becomes temporally organized. The craving appears "at that time" because the system has learned to expect a certain pattern there.

This timing specificity does not require dramatic conditioning theories to become meaningful. Human behavior naturally organizes around repeated patterns. Familiar transitions become psychologically efficient. Anticipated rewards become linked to recognizable contexts. The more stable the repetition, the easier the prediction becomes to activate later.

Routine strengthens specificity because routines reduce uncertainty. The nervous system often favors predictable associations. A familiar sequence can become rewarding partly because it creates continuity and expected structure. A particular food, beverage, sensory experience, or ritual may therefore become linked not only to the object itself, but to the transition surrounding it. The craving becomes attached to completion of the pattern.

This is why cravings sometimes feel connected to moments rather than purely to intake. The signal may emerge during a pause, a commute, a recovery period after stress, a familiar entertainment environment, or a repeated social setting. The craving is shaped not only by the object but by the surrounding structure.

Emotional states can also contribute to specificity. This does not mean every craving is "emotional eating," nor does it mean emotions are the sole explanation for food-related behavior. Emotional states are better understood as contexts that influence reward prediction. Stress, boredom, fatigue, loneliness, frustration, anxiety, restlessness, celebration, relief, and emotional depletion can all alter which rewards feel most available or most salient.

Under emotional strain, a previously reinforced sensory pattern may become more attractive because the system predicts regulation, interruption, familiarity, or relief. Under boredom, stimulation may become more valuable. Under fatigue, convenience and rapid accessibility may become more salient. Under loneliness, familiarity and comfort may gain psychological weight. Under celebration, reward intensity may become socially reinforced. The emotional state changes the meaning of the expected outcome.

Importantly, emotional specificity does not make cravings irrational. The system is not generating random impulses disconnected from context. It is organizing prediction around anticipated effects. The emotional state becomes part of the signal environment.

Environmental specificity further strengthens this process. Physical setting influences salience because the nervous system continuously evaluates cues associated with prior reward. Smell, lighting, packaging visibility, screen exposure, storage location, social atmosphere, sound, advertising, environmental repetition, and simple availability can all increase the accessibility of a specific craving.

The environment does not mechanically force behavior, but it shapes prediction. A cue associated with repeated reward may activate anticipation before conscious analysis occurs. The specificity of the craving therefore reflects not only internal state, but environmental memory.

Certain places become associated with certain expected outcomes. Certain activities become linked with certain sensory experiences. The context helps organize the direction of the signal.

Again, this is not an argument for fear-based environmental control. The purpose is interpretation, not behavioral instruction. The significance of environmental specificity is that it reveals how cravings become structured through repeated association. The system learns relevance from exposure patterns.

Memory contributes heavily to specificity because remembered reward remains psychologically available long after the original experience ends. The nervous system stores associations between sensory patterns and expected outcomes. A remembered experience of comfort, stimulation, relief, pleasure, familiarity, or decompression can later influence prediction even without immediate deprivation.

This is one reason cravings can arise suddenly in response to seemingly small cues. The cue may activate a larger predictive network involving memory, emotional context, timing pattern, and expected effect. The resulting craving may feel immediate, but the underlying structure has often been built gradually across repetition.

Specificity therefore reveals learned prediction. The signal narrows because the anticipated outcome has become organized around particular features. The craving points toward a target because the system predicts value there.

This prediction process becomes stronger under conditions of elevated pressure. Hunger, fatigue, stress load, sleep debt, unstable energy availability, emotional strain, and recovery limitation can all increase the intensity of specificity. The craving target may feel more urgent because broader system pressures amplify the reward prediction. The specificity becomes sharper under strain.

A fatigued system may narrow more quickly toward convenience, stimulation, or familiarity. A stressed system may assign greater value to relief-associated sensory patterns. Hunger may increase the urgency surrounding rapidly rewarding foods. Sleep debt may increase sensitivity to reward cues while reducing regulatory flexibility. These conditions do not create every craving, but they can increase the intensity of the predicted outcome.

The important point is that amplification and specificity interact. The craving becomes more compelling not simply because the target exists, but because the system is assigning greater predicted value to the target under current conditions.

This interaction helps explain why the same person may experience dramatically different craving intensity toward the same object across different states. The food itself did not suddenly become morally more powerful. The surrounding system conditions changed. Internal pressure, emotional context, fatigue state, environmental cues, timing patterns, and learned prediction shifted the perceived relevance of the target.

Specificity is therefore not evidence of weakness. It is evidence of organization.

The craving narrows because prediction narrows. The system identifies certain sensory and contextual patterns as especially associated with reward, regulation, familiarity, relief, or completion. That narrowing process can feel highly persuasive because concentrated predictions naturally command more attention than diffuse possibilities.

But concentrated attention is not proof of necessity.

A specific craving may feel meaningful because the anticipated outcome carries emotional or physiological salience. Yet the specificity itself primarily reveals learned association. The system predicts value based on previous experience, repeated context, and expected effect. The target becomes psychologically prioritized because prediction has become structured around it.

This distinction allows specificity to be interpreted without moralization. The craving does not need to be treated as evidence that the person lacks discipline. The specificity does not mean the food is inherently dangerous. It does not mean the person is "addicted" in a simplistic sense. It means the nervous system has organized reward prediction around a recognizable pattern.

That pattern may include texture, flavor, convenience, timing, emotional state, routine, environment, memory, or sensory familiarity. Often it includes several at once. The resulting signal feels directed because the prediction itself is directed.

The more clearly specificity is understood, the less mysterious cravings become. A craving that appears highly selective no longer needs to be interpreted as irrational weakness or biological destiny. The specificity can instead be read as a clue to the structure of the signal. The system has learned associations between certain targets and certain expected outcomes. The craving narrows because the prediction narrows.

Seen this way, specificity becomes interpretive information rather than moral evidence. The useful question is not why the person is unable to resist a specific craving. The more useful interpretation is that the system has organized reward expectation around a learned sensory and contextual pattern. The craving has direction because prediction has direction.

That direction may be shaped by familiarity, convenience, timing, emotional state, environmental exposure, repeated routines, remembered relief, sensory intensity, or anticipated regulation. The signal becomes specific because the system expects a specific effect.

Reward Expectation Mechanism

Cravings often become powerful before anything is consumed. The intensity appears early. The mind begins organizing around the anticipated response before the response itself occurs. Attention narrows. The target becomes more salient. The expected outcome begins to feel increasingly important. This sequence matters because it reveals that craving is not only directed toward an object. It is directed toward what the object is expected to produce.

A craving may therefore involve more than anticipation of taste or sensory pleasure. The system may be anticipating relief from discomfort, restoration of energy, emotional softening, familiarity, stimulation, regulation, completion of a routine, interruption of fatigue, or reduction of internal tension. The craving gains force because the expected state change becomes psychologically active before the outcome itself exists.

This is the Reward Expectation Mechanism.

The Reward Expectation Mechanism describes the process by which craving gains urgency because the system anticipates a future state change before the response occurs. The craving intensifies not only because a specific object has become relevant, but because the system predicts that engagement with that object will alter the current condition in a meaningful way. The anticipated outcome becomes part of the signal itself.

This distinction changes the interpretation of craving. The signal is no longer simply "I want this." It becomes "this is expected to change how the current state feels." The craving therefore carries prediction inside it. The object matters partly because of the anticipated effect attached to it.

This predictive structure helps explain why cravings can feel persuasive before any physical outcome has appeared. The system begins assigning value in advance. A remembered sensory pattern, environmental cue, emotional state, or internal pressure can activate anticipation before action occurs. The expected relief, pleasure, stimulation, comfort, or regulation becomes psychologically available before the actual experience exists.

The anticipation itself increases salience.

A person may therefore feel pulled toward a particular response long before the response has produced any concrete effect. The imagined outcome begins influencing behavior in advance. The system starts organizing around prediction rather than only around present conditions. Craving becomes future-oriented.

This future orientation is important because anticipated reward often feels emotionally cleaner and more complete than the eventual outcome itself. Before the response occurs, the predicted effect may appear especially convincing. The anticipated comfort may feel total. The expected pleasure may feel uncomplicated. The imagined relief may seem highly resolving. The craving therefore intensifies partly because the prediction becomes simplified and concentrated before reality introduces variability.

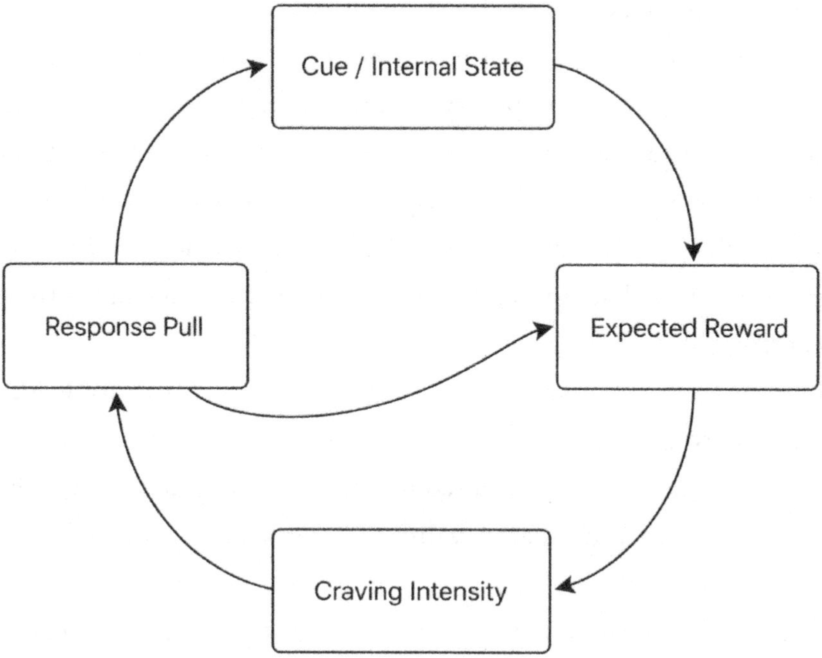

[Figure 4: Reward Expectation Loop]

The loop matters because expectation begins feeding urgency before the outcome exists. A cue or internal state activates anticipated reward. The anticipated reward increases craving intensity. The increased intensity increases behavioral pull. The behavioral pull reinforces future expectation. The process becomes self-strengthening because the predicted outcome gains psychological importance before the response itself fully unfolds.

This does not mean the expected outcome is imaginary. Many responses do produce pleasure, comfort, stimulation, relief, familiarity, or temporary regulation. The important distinction is not whether the reward exists. The important distinction is that anticipation and outcome are not identical experiences.

Anticipated relief often feels more complete than actual relief because prediction compresses complexity. Before the response occurs, the mind organizes around the expected shift in state rather than around the full range of possible outcomes. The expected change may feel singular and highly resolving. After the response occurs, the experience may become more mixed, partial, temporary, context-dependent, or less transformative than predicted.

This difference should not be interpreted morally. It is not evidence that the person was deceiving themselves or lacking insight. Prediction naturally simplifies expected outcomes because the system is organizing behavior around anticipated value. The expected reward becomes concentrated in advance.

A person may therefore experience a strong craving because the predicted effect feels unusually meaningful before action occurs. The anticipated comfort may feel emotionally important. The expected energy increase may feel necessary. The imagined relief may feel urgent. Once the response occurs, the actual experience may still contain reward, but the emotional intensity of anticipation may soften, fragment, or shift.

The gap between anticipation and outcome is structurally important because it helps explain why cravings can feel compelling even when prior experiences were inconsistent, partial, or short-lived. The system is not only recalling what happened previously. It is predicting what might happen next. Prediction organizes motivation around expected value rather than around objective certainty.

Pleasure is one expected outcome that can intensify craving, but pleasure alone does not explain the full structure of reward expectation. Many cravings involve anticipated regulation rather than simple enjoyment. The system may expect reduction of tension, interruption of fatigue, emotional softening, restoration of familiarity, temporary escape from discomfort, or stimulation during states of depletion or boredom.

Energy can become part of the expected outcome when the system associates a particular response with activation, alertness, or increased functional capacity. Under fatigue or cognitive strain, the anticipated effect may become more psychologically important because the current state already feels narrowed or depleted. The craving gains urgency because the expected state change feels relevant to immediate functioning.

Comfort functions similarly. A familiar sensory pattern may become associated with emotional settling, decompression, warmth, slowing down, or relief from pressure. The craving therefore becomes attached not only to taste, texture, or intake, but to the expected shift in emotional atmosphere. The anticipated comfort becomes part of the signal before the response occurs.

Regulation is another important dimension of reward expectation. A craving may intensify because the system predicts stabilization, grounding, interruption of agitation, or temporary reduction of internal friction. Again, this does not require dramatic language about addiction or pathology. Human systems continuously move toward predicted regulation. When a particular response becomes associated with perceived stabilization, anticipation itself can increase motivational pull.

Familiarity also matters. Familiar experiences often carry lower uncertainty and greater psychological predictability. A repeated sensory pattern may therefore become rewarding partly because it represents continuity. The expected familiarity reduces unpredictability. Under stress, fatigue, emotional strain, or cognitive overload, familiar responses may gain salience because the system assigns value to predictable outcomes.

Stimulation can operate in the opposite direction while following the same structural logic. Under boredom, low activation, monotony, or emotional flatness, the system may assign value to intensity, novelty, sensory engagement, or rapid state change. The craving intensifies because the expected effect appears capable of altering the present condition quickly.

These anticipated outcomes do not need to be consciously articulated in order to influence craving intensity. A person may not explicitly think, “I expect this to regulate my emotional state.” The predictive structure can operate implicitly. The body and brain continuously organize around expected outcomes without requiring constant verbal awareness. The craving therefore feels immediate even when the underlying prediction remains largely unspoken.

This helps explain why cravings often feel convincing before any external event occurs. The expected state change is already emotionally active inside the signal. The system is not merely remembering an object. It is simulating a future condition associated with that object. The anticipated future becomes motivationally relevant in the present.

Prediction becomes especially powerful under conditions of elevated internal pressure. Hunger, fatigue, stress load, sleep debt, emotional strain, unstable energy availability, or recovery limitation can increase the salience of expected reward because the system is already operating under strain. When the present state feels difficult, the anticipated state change becomes more behaviorally important.

Under these conditions, the predicted outcome may appear unusually valuable. Relief feels more urgent when tension is high. Stimulation feels more important when fatigue is heavy. Familiarity feels more meaningful when uncertainty increases. Comfort feels more persuasive when emotional strain accumulates. The current state alters the value assigned to the anticipated future state.

This is why cravings can intensify dramatically during periods of exhaustion, stress, instability, or emotional overload. The specific object does not necessarily become objectively more rewarding. The expected effect becomes more relevant because the system is already under pressure.

Reward expectation gains strength through contrast with the current condition.

The stronger the predicted state change, the stronger the behavioral pull can become.

This does not mean the system is irrational. Movement toward predicted reward is structurally understandable. Organisms naturally orient toward expected outcomes associated with relief, regulation, energy availability, familiarity, pleasure, or stabilization. The nervous system continuously prioritizes what appears relevant to reducing strain or improving state conditions.

Craving therefore becomes easier to understand when interpreted as predictive organization rather than simple indulgence. The system is attempting to move toward an anticipated outcome that appears meaningful under current conditions. The urgency reflects predicted value.

Importantly, expected reward is not inherently false. Sometimes the anticipated comfort genuinely occurs. Sometimes the response does produce pleasure, regulation, stimulation, familiarity, or temporary relief. The issue is not whether the expected outcome exists. The issue is that anticipation itself can become highly persuasive before the outcome unfolds fully.

The predictive state may therefore become stronger than the eventual physical effect. Anticipation concentrates attention around possibility. The imagined outcome may feel unusually clear because competing information temporarily fades into the background. Once the response occurs, the actual experience re-enters a more complex reality involving duration, adaptation, emotional context, changing physiology, and incomplete resolution.

This difference between anticipation and outcome helps explain why cravings can recur even after prior responses were imperfect. Prediction renews itself around expected value rather than relying solely on prior satisfaction. The anticipated future state continues carrying motivational weight.

Memory strengthens this process because remembered reward becomes emotionally accessible even when the original experience has passed. The system stores associations between specific responses and expected effects. A cue linked with prior pleasure, comfort, stimulation, or regulation can therefore reactivate anticipation later. The craving gains urgency because the expected outcome becomes psychologically available again.

The specificity of craving becomes important here because prediction is rarely abstract. The expected reward often becomes attached to a particular sensory profile, timing pattern, emotional context, environment, or routine. The craving narrows because the anticipated outcome has become associated with recognizable features. The system predicts not only reward in general, but reward through a specific pathway.

A familiar evening routine may therefore activate anticipated decompression before any response occurs. A stress-related context may activate anticipated relief. A fatigue state may activate anticipated stimulation. A lonely environment may activate anticipated comfort or familiarity. The craving becomes context-sensitive because prediction itself is context-sensitive.

Reward expectation also explains why cravings can feel emotionally disproportionate relative to the object itself. The intensity is not always about the sensory target alone. It may reflect the psychological importance assigned to the anticipated state change. The craving feels large because the expected outcome feels meaningful under current conditions.

Again, this does not require moral interpretation. A strong prediction is not evidence of weak character. It reflects the interaction between internal state, learned association, anticipated reward, and current pressure conditions. The craving becomes persuasive because the system expects relevance.

Understanding reward expectation changes how craving intensity is interpreted. Instead of assuming the person simply lacks discipline or “wants food too much,” the signal can be understood as future-oriented state prediction. The craving is carrying an anticipated outcome inside it. The system believes something important may happen if the response occurs.

That anticipated importance may involve pleasure, comfort, energy, familiarity, stimulation, regulation, or temporary reduction of discomfort. The expected effect organizes attention and increases urgency before the outcome exists. The craving becomes more understandable once it is interpreted as prediction rather than mere impulse.

A predicted effect can be meaningful without being complete.

Seen through this frame, craving is not only attraction to an object. It is movement toward an expected internal condition. The signal says more than “I want that.” Often, beneath the surface, the signal is communicating something closer to “that is expected to change how this state feels.”

The behavioral pull gains force because the anticipated future state already feels psychologically active in the present.

Dopamine Prediction Mechanism

Dopamine is frequently discussed in language that is both overly simplified and overly dramatic. It is often presented as a pleasure chemical, a reward switch, a hidden force behind every modern behavior, or the primary explanation for craving itself. In popular discussion, dopamine sometimes becomes shorthand for excess desire, overstimulation, compulsive behavior, distraction, or failed self-control. The resulting interpretation tends to flatten a complex motivational system into a single chemical story.

This framing creates confusion because it treats dopamine as though it were identical to pleasure. In reality, craving often intensifies before pleasure occurs. The signal becomes strong before the reward is experienced. Attention narrows before consumption. Motivational pull increases before satisfaction appears. The sequence itself suggests that craving cannot be explained by pleasure alone.

A more useful interpretation places dopamine-related signaling within prediction, salience, pursuit, learning, and reinforcement.

This is the Dopamine Prediction Mechanism.

The Dopamine Prediction Mechanism describes the process by which dopamine-related signaling helps assign importance to predicted reward, increases salience around relevant cues, supports motivational pursuit, and strengthens learned associations without being reducible to pleasure alone. Within craving, dopamine-related activity helps organize movement toward expected outcomes. It increases the relevance of certain possibilities before those possibilities become reality.

This distinction matters because the system often becomes activated around anticipated reward rather than around reward already obtained. The craving gains force before the outcome occurs because prediction itself becomes motivationally important. The nervous system begins prioritizing what appears likely to produce relief, comfort, stimulation, familiarity, regulation, energy, or other meaningful state changes.

Under this framework, dopamine-related signaling is less about passive enjoyment and more about active orientation. Certain cues become more noticeable. Certain expected outcomes become more psychologically important. Certain behaviors gain motivational weight. The system begins moving toward what it predicts may matter.

Oversimplified View	Systems View
Dopamine = Pleasure	Dopamine supports Prediction Salience Motivation Pursuit Reinforcement

[Figure 5: Dopamine Prediction Model]

The systems view changes interpretation significantly. If dopamine is reduced to pleasure alone, craving becomes difficult to explain accurately. A person may experience intense craving before any pleasure has occurred.

A cue may become highly motivating before the anticipated response happens. The object may gain urgency while still remaining entirely future-oriented. The signal is being strengthened by prediction and motivational relevance rather than by present enjoyment.

This helps explain why cravings can become focused and behaviorally persuasive in advance. The nervous system continuously evaluates which signals deserve attention, energy, and pursuit. Dopamine-related signaling participates in assigning salience to predicted reward opportunities. Salience means importance. A salient cue becomes harder to ignore because the system treats it as relevant to anticipated value.

A familiar food cue under conditions of fatigue, stress, emotional strain, or hunger may therefore become unusually noticeable. The object appears to stand out. Attention narrows toward it. The expected outcome becomes psychologically amplified. This process does not require the reward to be currently happening. Prediction alone can increase motivational pull.

The distinction between wanting and liking becomes useful here.

Wanting refers to the motivational pull toward an anticipated reward. Liking refers to the actual pleasurable experience or satisfaction associated with the reward itself. These experiences often overlap, but they are not identical. A person can strongly want something while experiencing only moderate satisfaction once it occurs. A person can enjoy something greatly without having experienced strong craving beforehand.

The difference matters because craving intensity is often more closely tied to wanting than to liking. The system may become highly activated around pursuit even when the eventual reward is partial, brief, inconsistent, or less satisfying than anticipated. The motivational force develops in advance because prediction and salience are already active.

This helps explain why cravings can feel persuasive even when previous experiences were imperfect. The system is not only remembering the final outcome. It is responding to anticipated possibility. Prediction renews motivational pull around expected reward rather than relying entirely on past satisfaction levels.

A craving therefore does not simply mean "this will feel good." More often, the signal carries something closer to "this is expected to matter." The predicted outcome gains importance under current conditions. The system assigns priority accordingly.

This assignment of priority is adaptive in principle. Organisms must continuously orient toward predicted opportunities related to energy, safety, regulation, learning, comfort, social connection, or relief from strain. Dopamine-related signaling participates in helping the nervous system identify what appears behaviorally relevant. Without predictive motivation, learning and adaptive pursuit would become difficult.

The problem with oversimplified dopamine narratives is that they often treat normal motivational processes as inherently pathological. Craving becomes interpreted as chemical hijacking rather than as amplified prediction within a broader system. The result is frequently unnecessary moralization or fear surrounding ordinary human reward processes.

Dopamine-related signaling is not a villain inside the nervous system. It is part of how the system learns what matters, what predicts value, and what deserves attention or pursuit. The existence of motivational pull does not prove weakness or dysfunction. It reflects a predictive organism attempting to organize behavior around anticipated outcomes.

This becomes especially relevant when cravings intensify under conditions of internal pressure. Hunger, fatigue, emotional strain, stress load, glucose instability, sleep debt, under-recovery, and prolonged cognitive demand can all increase the salience of expected reward. When the present state feels strained, the predicted value of relief, comfort, stimulation, familiarity, or rapid regulation becomes more behaviorally important.

Under these conditions, dopamine-related signaling may help increase the motivational relevance of cues associated with anticipated improvement. A fatigued person may become more sensitive to signals predicting energy or stimulation. A stressed person may become more responsive to cues associated with relief or decompression. A lonely or emotionally strained person may experience stronger pull toward familiarity, comfort, or emotionally meaningful routines.

Again, dopamine is not replacing the system in these situations. It is participating within it. The motivational pull emerges from interaction between internal state, expected reward, learned association, cue exposure, memory, and current pressure conditions. Dopamine-related signaling helps organize salience and pursuit inside that larger network.

This broader frame prevents reductionism.

Craving is not "just dopamine." Appetite pressure matters. Sleep state matters. Fatigue matters. Emotional strain matters. Environmental exposure matters. Timing patterns matter. Repetition matters. Learned associations matter. Glucose variability, stress load, familiarity, availability, and memory all contribute to how strongly a signal becomes amplified. Dopamine-related processes participate in shaping motivational relevance within this larger structure, but they do not replace the structure itself.

Reductionist explanations often fail because they collapse multi-layered experiences into a single mechanism. Human craving does not emerge from one isolated variable. It develops through interaction between physiology, prediction, memory, context, reinforcement, and current state conditions. Dopamine-related signaling becomes meaningful when understood as one layer supporting prediction and motivational organization rather than as a total explanation.

Prediction remains central because the nervous system continuously evaluates future-oriented possibilities. A cue associated with prior reward can become motivationally significant before any outcome occurs. The cue gains power because the system expects something relevant to follow from it. Dopamine-related signaling helps support this predictive orientation by increasing salience around anticipated opportunity.

This is why cues matter so strongly in craving. The object itself is not the entire signal. The cue activates prediction of a future state change. The anticipated outcome becomes emotionally and behaviorally active before the reward arrives. The craving therefore gains urgency because expected reward is already psychologically present in partial form.

The specificity of craving further supports this process. Cravings often attach to particular textures, environments, times of day, routines, emotional states, sensory profiles, or remembered effects because prediction becomes organized around learned associations. The nervous system learns that certain cues tend to precede certain outcomes. Over time, the cue itself acquires motivational relevance.

A familiar evening environment may therefore increase salience around anticipated decompression. A repeated stress context may increase attention toward cues associated with comfort or relief. A fatigue state may heighten sensitivity toward stimulation-associated rewards. The cue becomes more than a neutral object because prediction has linked it to anticipated state change.

Reinforcement contributes to this learning process. When cues, cravings, responses, and rewarding or regulating outcomes become repeatedly associated, the nervous system becomes more efficient at recognizing and prioritizing those associations later. Dopamine-related prediction helps strengthen the connection between anticipated reward and relevant cues.

This does not require dramatic language about addiction or permanent rewiring. Reinforcement is a normal feature of learning systems. Repeatedly paired experiences become easier to recognize and predict. The system becomes increasingly prepared to respond to familiar patterns.

The strengthening of association can increase craving intensity because future cues begin activating motivational pull more quickly. The anticipated reward becomes more accessible. The signal gains efficiency. Certain environments, routines, emotional states, or sensory patterns become increasingly capable of triggering pursuit before conscious deliberation fully develops.

Again, the important point is not that dopamine creates every craving. The important point is that dopamine-related signaling helps support predictive relevance and motivational orientation within a larger reinforcement system.

The wanting-versus-liking distinction becomes particularly important here because reinforcement can strengthen pursuit even when satisfaction remains inconsistent. The system may continue assigning motivational importance to predicted reward despite variability in actual enjoyment. The anticipation itself remains behaviorally powerful.

This explains why craving intensity cannot be measured simply by asking how pleasurable the final experience was. The pursuit process has its own motivational structure. Prediction can remain compelling even when outcomes fluctuate. The expected possibility continues generating salience and wanting.

Importantly, this does not mean people are trapped by dopamine-driven behavior. The chapter is not arguing for inevitability, helplessness, or biological determinism. It is clarifying how motivational systems organize around anticipated relevance. Understanding prediction and salience improves interpretation without requiring moral panic or simplistic control narratives.

This also prevents dopamine from becoming a cultural shorthand for excess stimulation itself. Modern discussions sometimes treat dopamine as though it were inherently dangerous whenever reward becomes intense or frequent. But dopamine-related signaling participates in ordinary learning, curiosity, motivation, exploration, attachment, pursuit, and adaptation. The existence of dopamine involvement does not automatically transform an experience into pathology.

The more useful question is not whether dopamine is involved. Dopamine-related processes are involved in many forms of motivated behavior. The more useful question is how prediction, internal state, repetition, learned association, and current pressure conditions are shaping salience and behavioral pull.

A craving therefore becomes easier to interpret once dopamine is repositioned away from pleasure absolutism. The signal is not merely a chemical command for enjoyment. It is a predictive motivational process shaped by expected relevance. The craving gains force because the system believes something meaningful may follow from the anticipated response.

That expected relevance may involve pleasure, comfort, regulation, stimulation, familiarity, relief, energy, or interruption of strain. Dopamine-related signaling helps make those anticipated outcomes more noticeable and motivationally important before they occur.

Seen through this lens, craving becomes less mysterious and less moralized. The intensity is not proof of weak character, nor is it proof that one neurotransmitter has taken over the system. The craving reflects predictive salience operating within a broader network of reinforcement, internal pressure, memory, environmental exposure, repetition, and expected reward.

Dopamine becomes most useful when understood as part of how the system learns what to pursue, what to notice, and what to predict as meaningful. The signal gains motivational force before reward arrives because prediction itself has become behaviorally important.

Anticipation Pressure Mechanism

Craving often develops through a buildup phase before any response occurs. The signal may begin quietly as a passing image, remembered sensory detail, environmental cue, emotional association, or vague expectation. At first, the pull may feel mild. The target appears briefly in awareness, then recedes. But if attention returns repeatedly to the anticipated outcome, the signal can intensify. The craving becomes more organized, more urgent, and more behaviorally significant before anything has been consumed.

This sequence matters because the increase in pressure often occurs before any physical change has taken place. The body may not be more depleted than it was several minutes earlier. Energy availability may not have changed meaningfully. Hunger may not have intensified. Yet the craving itself becomes stronger. The buildup is being driven not only by biological need, but by anticipation.

The system begins organizing around an expected outcome.

A remembered reward becomes mentally available. The anticipated state change becomes more vivid. Attention narrows around the possibility of relief, comfort, stimulation, familiarity, pleasure, regulation, or interruption of discomfort. The predicted reward begins occupying more psychological space. As this process continues, wanting can intensify before the reward itself exists.

This is the Anticipation Pressure Mechanism.

The Anticipation Pressure Mechanism describes the process by which craving pressure rises before response as predicted reward becomes more salient, attention narrows around the expected outcome, and the anticipated state change begins to feel increasingly necessary. The pressure develops because the system is orienting toward a predicted future condition. The anticipated reward gains motivational weight before the outcome occurs physically.

This buildup helps explain why cravings can feel disproportionately urgent relative to immediate biological conditions. The intensity may not reflect increasing physical depletion. Instead, it may reflect increasing psychological organization around the expected outcome. The anticipated reward becomes more central. The signal gains pressure because prediction gains importance.

Craving therefore does not always arrive fully formed. It often accumulates.

A cue may activate a remembered possibility. The remembered possibility may reactivate expected relief or stimulation. The expected effect may increase attention toward the target. The increased attention may strengthen anticipation. The anticipation may increase motivational pull. The signal gradually becomes louder because the system keeps returning to the predicted outcome.

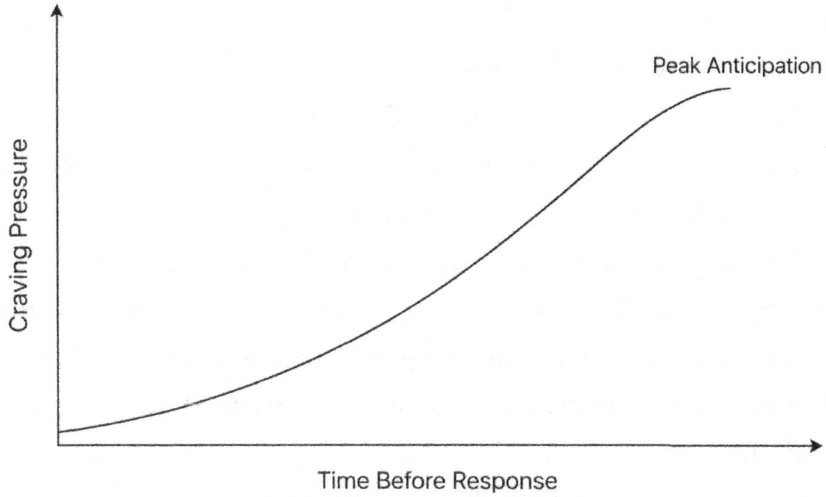

[Figure 6: Anticipation Pressure Curve]

The curve is important because it illustrates that wanting can intensify before reward is received. The rise in craving pressure occurs during the buildup itself. The anticipated outcome becomes increasingly salient as the predicted response approaches. The peak intensity may therefore occur before consumption rather than during it.

This process is often misunderstood because people assume urgency must reflect immediate need. But anticipation pressure can rise even when biological conditions remain relatively stable. A person may not be physically more depleted, yet the craving may become more difficult to ignore. The increase in pressure reflects prediction and salience rather than sudden worsening of physical need.

This distinction helps explain urgency without depletion.

A craving may intensify because the anticipated outcome feels psychologically closer and increasingly important. Relief appears more available. Comfort feels more imaginable. Stimulation seems more immediate. Familiarity becomes more emotionally relevant. The expected state change begins exerting motivational pull before the state itself has changed.

The nervous system continuously prioritizes predicted opportunities according to expected relevance. When a particular response becomes associated with meaningful relief, regulation, stimulation, or comfort, anticipation itself can increase urgency. The system begins behaving as though the expected outcome deserves increasing priority.

This urgency can feel persuasive because anticipation narrows attention.

As craving pressure rises, competing information may become quieter. Other priorities remain present but lose salience relative to the anticipated reward. The expected outcome occupies more cognitive space. The target becomes easier to think about and harder to stop thinking about. Attention circles back repeatedly toward the prediction.

This narrowing does not necessarily occur because the object itself has become objectively more important. It occurs because the anticipated effect has become motivationally central. The system is assigning increasing relevance to the predicted state change.

A person experiencing anticipation pressure may therefore feel that the anticipated reward has become unusually necessary. The signal acquires emotional weight. The predicted outcome appears increasingly capable of changing the current condition. The craving intensifies because the expected shift in state feels increasingly meaningful.

This process is especially important because anticipation itself functions as a pressure state rather than merely as passive imagination.

Anticipation changes system orientation. The body and brain begin preparing around a possible future response. The expected reward becomes psychologically active before it exists physically. The system partially enters the future condition in predictive form. Relief is anticipated before relief arrives. Comfort is imagined before comfort occurs. Stimulation becomes emotionally available before stimulation is experienced directly.

This predictive activation helps explain why anticipation pressure can feel physically real even before any external action takes place. The craving is not only conceptual. It becomes motivationally embodied. Attention, emotional relevance, and behavioral orientation begin reorganizing around the expected outcome.

The buildup phase can therefore feel increasingly difficult to ignore not because the anticipated reward is objectively essential, but because prediction itself is becoming amplified.

Delay sometimes intensifies this process.

Delay does not always weaken craving. In some situations, delaying response creates additional time for anticipation to organize itself around the expected reward. The system continues returning to the prediction. The target becomes more vivid. The expected outcome becomes increasingly concentrated. Attention repeatedly cycles through imagined relief, comfort, stimulation, familiarity, or regulation.

As anticipation repeats, the craving may gain force because the predicted reward continues occupying motivational space without resolution. The signal remains active. The expected state change remains unfinished. The buildup continues.

This is important because many discussions of craving assume that intensity always fades naturally with time. In reality, anticipation pressure can move in multiple directions. Sometimes a craving decreases when attention shifts and prediction loses salience. Other times the craving intensifies because the anticipated outcome becomes increasingly central through repetition and mental return.

The point is not that delay inevitably strengthens craving. Anticipation pressure is not perfectly linear or universally predictable. The rise and fall of craving depends on multiple interacting conditions, including internal state, cue exposure, emotional context, environmental salience, repetition of attention, and expected reward value.

But delay can create conditions where anticipation gains additional structure. The system keeps orienting toward the unresolved prediction. The target becomes increasingly psychologically present. The expected outcome feels progressively more important because the anticipation itself remains active.

This helps explain why cravings can sometimes feel stronger after extended mental engagement with the anticipated reward than they did initially. The buildup creates pressure through continued prediction. The wanting becomes amplified through repeated orientation toward the expected outcome.

Importantly, anticipation pressure differs from actual reward.

The buildup phase is often driven more by wanting than by liking. The craving gains intensity before pleasure occurs. The system becomes highly organized around pursuit before satisfaction exists. The motivational pull therefore reflects anticipated value more than present enjoyment.

This distinction matters because anticipation can sometimes feel cleaner and more emotionally concentrated than the actual outcome. Before response occurs, the expected relief may seem highly complete. The anticipated comfort may feel unusually resolving. The imagined stimulation may appear especially meaningful. Once the response happens, the experience may become more mixed, temporary, partial, or variable than prediction suggested.

Again, this is not deception or failure. Prediction naturally simplifies anticipated outcomes because the system is organizing behavior around expected relevance. The anticipated future state becomes emotionally compressed into a concentrated motivational signal.

The buildup therefore acquires emotional intensity partly because anticipation reduces complexity. The expected outcome appears singular and psychologically important. Competing information becomes less salient. The craving feels persuasive because prediction has narrowed around one anticipated direction.

Internal pressure can amplify this narrowing significantly.

Hunger may increase the perceived value of anticipated intake. Fatigue may increase the appeal of stimulation, convenience, or rapid relief. Stress load may increase sensitivity toward comfort-associated rewards. Sleep debt may increase motivational pull toward familiar or quickly rewarding experiences. Emotional strain may increase the salience of anticipated soothing, interruption, or decompression. Glucose instability may increase urgency surrounding rapid state change or expected energy restoration.

These conditions do not create every craving, but they can intensify anticipation pressure because the current state already feels strained. The predicted reward becomes more psychologically valuable through contrast with the present condition.

When the system is under pressure, expected relief gains importance.

A fatigued person may experience stronger anticipation around stimulation because the present state feels heavy. A stressed person may experience stronger anticipation around comfort because emotional tension increases the value of predicted decompression. A hungry person may experience stronger anticipation around specific reward because appetite pressure amplifies expected satisfaction.

The craving therefore gains urgency partly because the anticipated state change appears capable of resolving something meaningful about the present condition.

This does not mean the anticipated reward is necessarily false. Sometimes the response genuinely does provide comfort, stimulation, familiarity, pleasure, regulation, or temporary relief. The important issue is that anticipation itself becomes motivationally active before the outcome exists. The buildup creates pressure in advance.

The system begins preparing around the predicted possibility.

This future-oriented organization is one reason cravings can feel so emotionally convincing. The anticipated outcome partially occupies the present before it physically occurs. The system behaves as though the predicted state already matters. The craving therefore feels urgent because prediction itself has become psychologically real.

Anticipation pressure also helps explain why cravings can fluctuate rapidly depending on salience conditions. The same object may feel mildly relevant in one moment and highly compelling in another. The difference often reflects changes in predictive organization rather than dramatic changes in biological necessity.

Environmental cues, emotional state, fatigue level, stress load, repeated attention, memory activation, and internal pressure all influence how strongly anticipation builds around a predicted outcome. The craving becomes more intense when the expected reward occupies greater motivational space.

This understanding changes interpretation significantly.

Without recognizing anticipation pressure, craving intensity can appear mysterious or morally loaded. The person may assume that strong urgency proves weakness, lack of discipline, or overwhelming need. But much of the intensity may belong to the buildup itself. The signal becomes amplified because prediction, salience, and attention narrowing are increasing pressure before any reward occurs.

Seen this way, anticipation becomes easier to interpret structurally. The craving is not merely announcing present biological necessity. It is organizing around expected future change. The buildup reflects motivational pressure created by anticipated reward.

The signal therefore says more than "I need this now." Often, beneath the surface, the signal is communicating something closer to "this is expected to change the current state in an important way."

The expected relief, comfort, stimulation, familiarity, energy, or regulation becomes increasingly psychologically central as anticipation intensifies. Attention narrows. Salience rises. The predicted reward feels more necessary than it may actually be.

This does not make the craving unreal. It makes the buildup interpretable.

The intensity belongs partly to the pressure created by prediction itself. The craving becomes more readable once anticipation is recognized not as passive imagination, but as an active motivational state shaped by expected reward, narrowing attention, and increasing salience before the outcome occurs.

Cue Association Mechanism

Cravings often appear to begin internally. A person suddenly thinks about a specific food, sensory experience, or anticipated reward, and the craving seems to emerge from nowhere. The experience feels spontaneous, personal, and immediate. But many cravings are activated before conscious choice fully forms. The initiating signal may arrive through ordinary context rather than deliberate intention. A familiar environment, repeated routine, emotional state, transition point, or sensory exposure can activate reward expectation before the person fully recognizes that the process has already begun.

This is one reason cravings can feel confusing. The cue that activated the signal is often familiar enough to disappear into the background. The person notices the craving but not always the pattern that brought the craving forward. The activation feels self-generated because the triggering conditions were ordinary, repeated, and structurally embedded into daily life.

Craving therefore does not always begin with deliberate desire. Often it begins with recognition.

The system encounters a familiar context associated with prior reward, relief, comfort, stimulation, familiarity, or regulation. Prediction becomes active. Salience increases. The expected outcome becomes psychologically available before conscious analysis fully catches up. The craving emerges because the nervous system recognizes a learned pattern.

This is the Cue Association Mechanism.

The Cue Association Mechanism describes the process by which repeated pairings between cues and expected reward teach the system to activate craving when familiar contexts, sensations, routines, or internal states appear. The cue gains predictive relevance through repetition. Over time, the context itself begins helping initiate craving pressure because the expected outcome has become associated with recognizable conditions.

The important distinction is that cues do not force behavior. A cue is not a command. It is a prediction made visible.

The nervous system continuously evaluates the environment for patterns associated with meaningful outcomes. When a cue repeatedly appears alongside reward, comfort, relief, stimulation, regulation, or familiarity, the cue gradually becomes linked with expectation. The system learns that certain conditions tend to precede certain experiences. Once the association strengthens, the cue itself can begin activating anticipation before the response occurs.

This activation often happens quickly and quietly. A smell, location, emotional shift, transition in routine, visual exposure, or familiar timing pattern may increase salience without dramatic conscious awareness. The target becomes more noticeable. The expected reward becomes easier to imagine. The craving signal becomes more available.

Importantly, the cue does not need to be extraordinary. In many cases, the most powerful cues are structurally ordinary because repetition increases familiarity. Time of day can become predictive. Place can become predictive. Routines become predictive. Emotional states become predictive. Screens, sounds, lighting conditions, driving routes, post-work transitions, social settings, availability patterns, and repeated environmental exposures can all become linked to anticipated reward.

The system learns continuity between context and outcome.

Evening transition periods provide a useful structural example. A person may repeatedly pair the end of work with decompression, comfort, stimulation, reward, or interruption of cognitive strain. Over time, the transition itself becomes meaningful. The craving may begin appearing before hunger is especially strong because the system recognizes the familiar pattern. The anticipated outcome becomes psychologically available through the context alone.

The same process can occur during screen use, driving routes, social gatherings, weekend routines, after-dinner periods, or repeated entertainment environments. The craving becomes associated not only with the object itself, but with the sequence surrounding it. Context organizes prediction.

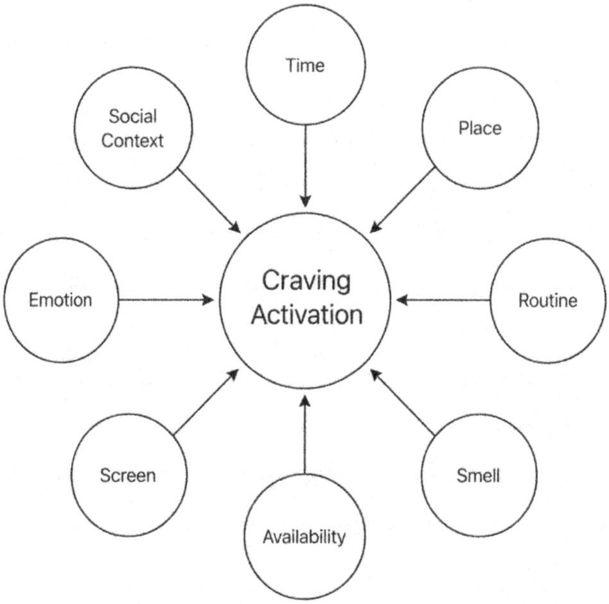

[Figure 7: Cue Activation Map]

The map matters because craving activation is often distributed across multiple cue layers at once. Time, place, routine, emotion, smell, screens, social atmosphere, availability, and internal state may all converge around the same expected reward. The resulting signal feels internally unified even though its activation emerged through multiple associations operating simultaneously.

A cue therefore functions less like a trigger in a mechanical sense and more like an activation point within a learned network of prediction. The cue increases accessibility. It helps bring anticipated reward into awareness. The system begins orienting toward a possible outcome because familiar conditions have appeared again.

Repeated exposure strengthens this process because familiarity increases predictive efficiency. The nervous system becomes faster at recognizing contexts associated with prior reward or regulation. Less conscious effort is required for anticipation to emerge. The cue gains psychological relevance through repetition.

A familiar environment can therefore activate craving before deliberate intention appears. The person may not initially decide to pursue reward. The environment itself may already be increasing salience around expected outcomes. Attention begins shifting toward the anticipated possibility before conscious planning fully forms.

This helps explain why cravings can arise in the absence of significant hunger. The system may not be broadly energy-depleted, yet the context itself activates prediction. The craving appears because the nervous system recognizes a familiar association rather than because biological need suddenly increased.

Context can therefore create craving before hunger appears.

This distinction is important because it prevents craving from being interpreted exclusively through energy need. A person may encounter a familiar cue pattern associated with comfort, decompression, stimulation, familiarity, or reward, and the craving becomes active even though broad intake relevance remains relatively unchanged. The activation reflects learned prediction more than immediate depletion.

A familiar cue does not create biological necessity. It increases anticipated relevance.

Time-of-day patterns illustrate this clearly because repeated rhythms become psychologically organized over time. Evening may become associated with emotional release after sustained effort. Weekend environments may become associated with loosened structure and anticipated reward. Certain commuting patterns may become associated with transition out of responsibility and into comfort. A post-meal period may become associated with completion rituals or expected sensory continuation.

The clock itself is not causing craving. The timing represents accumulated association.

This is equally true for place-based patterns. Certain rooms, seating arrangements, stores, entertainment settings, restaurants, or social environments become associated with expected outcomes because they repeatedly accompany reward-related experiences. Entering the environment increases salience because the nervous system recognizes the familiar structure.

Memory strengthens these associations further. The cue not only signals present context. It also activates remembered outcomes connected to previous experiences. A familiar smell, sound, or visual pattern can reactivate emotional and sensory expectation quickly because the system stores associations between context and predicted reward.

The cue therefore functions as a bridge between present environment and anticipated future state.

Smell often becomes especially powerful because sensory memory is highly associative. A familiar scent linked with comfort, pleasure, warmth, stimulation, or familiarity may rapidly activate anticipated reward before conscious analysis fully develops. Again, this is not because smell overrides agency. It is because sensory cues can efficiently activate learned prediction networks.

Visual exposure operates similarly. Repeated pairing between certain images and expected outcomes increases salience when those images reappear. Packaging, advertising, screens, entertainment environments, and repeated visual contexts can therefore increase craving availability because they reactivate anticipated reward associations.

A repeated cue becomes easier for the system to recognize. Recognition increases prediction. Prediction increases salience.

Internal states function as cues as well.

Craving is often discussed as though it were activated only by external environment, but emotional and physiological conditions can become predictive contexts in their own right. Stress, fatigue, boredom, loneliness, restlessness, cognitive overload, emotional strain, frustration, and under-recovery can all become associated with anticipated reward if they repeatedly precede certain forms of relief-seeking or regulation-seeking.

A fatigued state may therefore activate craving because the system has learned to associate exhaustion with anticipated stimulation, comfort, convenience, or decompression. Stress may activate craving because prior experiences linked stress with relief or interruption. Boredom may increase salience around stimulation-associated rewards. Emotional strain may increase motivational pull toward familiarity or soothing experiences.

The internal state becomes part of the cue structure.

This is important because it prevents cue association from being reduced to simplistic environmental explanations. The nervous system learns patterns across internal and external conditions simultaneously. A specific emotional atmosphere may become just as predictive as a physical location.

Availability also matters because accessible reward shortens the psychological distance between cue and expected outcome. When anticipated reward feels immediate and reachable, salience often increases. The possibility becomes easier to imagine concretely. The anticipated response gains motivational presence because the pathway toward it appears direct and available.

This does not mean availability determines behavior automatically. Availability modifies immediacy. A visible, familiar, easily accessible reward tends to become more psychologically active because the predicted outcome feels closer and more behaviorally relevant.

Again, the important point is interpretation rather than environmental control. The existence of cue association does not require fear of cues. Environments are not enemies. Familiarity is not failure. Human systems naturally learn predictive patterns across repeated contexts.

A learned cue is not weakness becoming visible. It is repetition becoming efficient.

This distinction matters because cravings are often moralized precisely at the moment when cue activation is strongest. The person experiences sudden wanting and assumes the craving emerged from defective character or failed discipline. But much of the activation may have occurred before conscious deliberation fully formed. The system recognized a familiar predictive structure and began organizing around expected reward.

That organization can happen quickly because repeated patterns reduce cognitive uncertainty. The nervous system favors efficiency. Familiar associations become easier to activate over time because the prediction pathway has already been practiced repeatedly.

This helps explain why some cravings feel immediate and emotionally convincing despite relatively stable physical conditions. The cue structure activates anticipated reward rapidly. The craving gains salience because the system already recognizes the pattern.

A cue does not create value from nothing. It activates remembered value attached to context.

The craving therefore becomes more understandable when interpreted as learned activation rather than spontaneous moral failure. The signal is being brought forward through association. The environment, timing pattern, emotional state, sensory exposure, or repeated routine is helping organize anticipation before deliberate choice fully develops.

Importantly, cue association remains flexible rather than perfectly fixed. Associations strengthen and weaken across changing conditions, repetition patterns, emotional contexts, physiological states, and environmental exposure. The system continuously updates prediction according to experience. Cue activation is dynamic rather than absolute.

This flexibility matters because it prevents deterministic interpretations. A learned association is not permanent destiny. It is a pattern of predictive relevance shaped through repetition and context. The nervous system continuously adapts according to what repeatedly appears meaningful.

Still, repeated pairings can create remarkably strong anticipatory activation because prediction becomes increasingly efficient. The cue begins carrying part of the reward expectation itself. The craving activates earlier in the sequence because the system already anticipates what may follow.

The buildup therefore starts before conscious pursuit fully forms.

This explains why cravings can sometimes feel surprisingly sudden even when they developed gradually through layered cue exposure. The activation sequence may have already been unfolding quietly through time, place, routine, emotional state, environmental familiarity, and anticipated reward before the craving became fully conscious.

Once recognized structurally, cue association becomes easier to interpret without moral distortion. The craving activated because the system encountered familiar predictive conditions. The response readiness reflects learned association between context and expected outcome.

The useful interpretation is not that the person failed a test of discipline. The more accurate interpretation is that the nervous system recognized a familiar pattern and began preparing for anticipated reward, relief, stimulation, comfort, familiarity, or regulation.

The signal becomes readable once the cue structure becomes visible.

Response Reinforcement Mechanism

Cravings become more powerful over time not only because they are experienced, but because they are repeatedly followed by responses that teach the system what to expect. A signal that repeatedly moves through the same sequence begins to organize itself more efficiently. The pathway becomes easier to recognize, easier to activate, and easier to repeat. Over time, the craving no longer feels like an isolated event. It becomes part of a learned loop.

This does not require conscious intention. The system continuously learns from repeated pairings between cue, anticipation, response, and outcome. When a familiar signal repeatedly produces a meaningful result, the sequence becomes increasingly available for future activation. The craving gains structure through repetition.

This is the Response Reinforcement Mechanism.

The Response Reinforcement Mechanism describes the process by which repeated pairing between cue, craving, response, and reward strengthens the likelihood, speed, intensity, and automaticity of future craving activation. The loop becomes more efficient because the nervous system learns the sequence and begins preparing for it earlier and more quickly.

Craving therefore becomes easier to activate when the pathway has been repeated many times. The cue becomes more recognizable. The anticipated outcome becomes more available. The response becomes more expected. The system develops readiness around the sequence itself.

The loop can be understood structurally:

Cue → Craving Signal → Response → Reward / Relief → Reinforcement

A cue appears. The cue activates prediction. The craving signal narrows attention around an anticipated outcome. A response follows. The response produces some form of meaningful result, whether pleasure, comfort, stimulation, familiarity, relief, regulation, interruption of discomfort, or reduction of tension. The system registers that the sequence led somewhere significant. Reinforcement strengthens future recognition of the pathway.

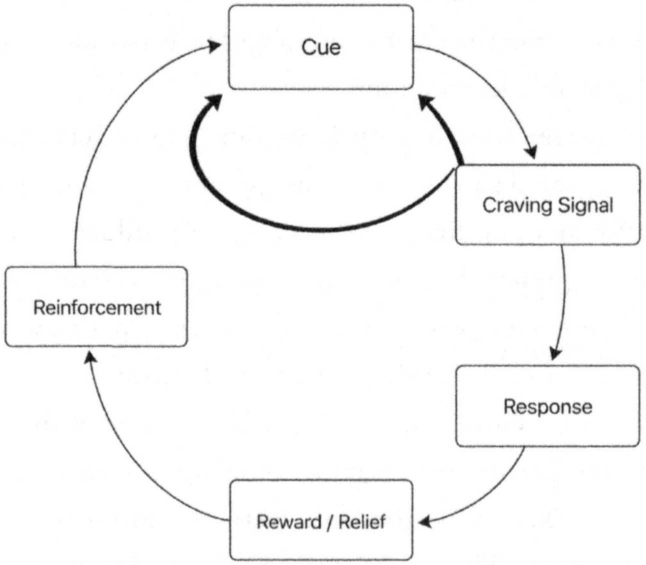

[Figure 8: Reinforced Signal Loop]

The reinforced loop matters because repetition changes efficiency. A pathway repeatedly associated with meaningful outcomes becomes easier for the nervous system to activate again. Less input may eventually be required to initiate the signal because the sequence has become familiar.

The cue is the entry point of the loop, but cues become meaningful only through repeated association. A particular time of day, environment, emotional state, transition period, sensory exposure, or internal condition begins activating anticipation because the system has repeatedly linked that condition with a rewarding or regulating outcome.

The craving signal then organizes attention around the expected effect. The signal becomes motivationally relevant because the anticipated outcome carries value. The expected reward does not need to be purely pleasurable. It may involve comfort, decompression, emotional interruption, familiarity, stimulation, regulation, or relief from internal pressure. The craving gains force because the system predicts significance.

The response follows the activation. The person moves toward the anticipated outcome. The outcome itself may vary in intensity or duration, but if the system registers the sequence as meaningful, the pathway becomes easier to recognize and prepare for later.

Reinforcement occurs because the nervous system learns from repeated pairings. The system updates prediction according to repeated experience. A sequence that repeatedly produces reward or relief gains psychological efficiency over time.

Repetition does not prove weakness. It proves the system has learned the sequence.

This distinction matters because reinforcement is often interpreted morally rather than structurally. Repeated cravings are frequently treated as evidence that the person lacks discipline, possesses poor character, or has failed repeatedly in some personal way. But reinforcement is not indictment. Reinforcement is learning.

The nervous system is designed to recognize patterns associated with meaningful outcomes. When a cue repeatedly predicts a valued result, the pathway becomes increasingly efficient. The system prepares earlier because prior experience taught it that preparation may be useful.

A repeated loop becomes faster because prediction becomes faster.

The sequence gradually requires less conscious assembly. The cue no longer needs to be analyzed in detail each time because the association already exists. The system recognizes the pattern quickly and begins activating anticipation before conscious deliberation fully forms.

This is where automaticity begins to matter.

Automaticity does not mean loss of agency or robotic behavior. It means the sequence becomes easier and quicker to activate because repetition reduces uncertainty. Familiar patterns require less cognitive effort for recognition. The cue begins activating readiness more rapidly because the nervous system already understands the expected structure.

A familiar environment may therefore produce craving almost immediately, not because the person has no choice, but because the sequence has become highly efficient through repetition. The system recognizes the pattern and begins organizing around the anticipated outcome before extensive conscious reflection occurs.

The loop becomes compressed.

This compression changes timing. Earlier in the learning process, the cue may have produced only mild interest or vague awareness. After repeated pairings, the same cue may produce stronger salience, quicker anticipation, and more immediate motivational pull. The signal intensifies because the pathway has become increasingly organized.

A learned loop reduces the distance between cue and expectation.

This helps explain why repeated craving patterns can feel increasingly automatic over time. The system becomes more efficient at predicting what comes next. The expected reward becomes more mentally available.

Attention narrows more quickly. The anticipated outcome gains salience earlier in the sequence.

Importantly, the strengthening of the pathway does not require the outcome to be perfect every time. Reinforcement does not depend on flawless satisfaction. The system learns from repeated meaningful associations even when outcomes vary. The anticipated reward may remain behaviorally relevant because the sequence has repeatedly produced some form of significance, relief, stimulation, familiarity, or regulation.

This is one reason craving loops can remain powerful even when the final outcome is mixed, partial, temporary, or inconsistent. Prediction and reinforcement are organized around meaningful possibility, not only around perfect satisfaction.

The lowering of activation threshold becomes especially important here.

An activation threshold refers to how much input is required before the signal becomes active. Early in a reinforcement process, a stronger or more direct cue may be necessary to initiate craving. Over time, repeated pairings can lower the threshold required for activation. Smaller cues become sufficient because the pathway has become increasingly sensitive to recognition.

A mild environmental reminder may eventually activate strong anticipation because the system already understands the sequence. A subtle emotional shift may become enough to initiate craving because the internal state has repeatedly preceded reward-seeking. A familiar transition point may trigger response readiness quickly because the nervous system has learned the pattern thoroughly.

Less activation becomes necessary once the pathway becomes efficient.

This does not mean the person becomes permanently trapped inside reinforcement loops. It means the system becomes skilled at recognizing repeated structures. The nervous system naturally increases efficiency around patterns associated with meaningful outcomes.

Efficiency itself is not pathology.

The same learning processes support language acquisition, social familiarity, routine coordination, skill development, and environmental adaptation. Reinforcement becomes concerning only when interpreted narrowly through moral judgment or simplistic self-control narratives. In reality, reinforcement reflects the nervous system's basic capacity to learn from repetition.

The structure of the craving loop also explains why reinforcement can involve relief as much as pleasure.

A response does not need to feel intensely pleasurable in order to strengthen the pathway. Reduction of discomfort, interruption of stress, softening of emotional strain, temporary quieting of agitation, restoration of familiarity, or movement away from internal pressure can all contribute to reinforcement. The system learns not only from positive reward, but from meaningful state change.

Relief can strengthen repetition because the nervous system registers reduction of discomfort as significant.

This distinction matters because many craving patterns are not organized solely around pleasure-seeking. Some become reinforced because the response consistently alters an unwanted condition. A fatigued state may become linked with stimulation-seeking. A stressed state may become linked with decompression routines. Emotional strain may become linked with comfort-associated sensory experiences. The pathway strengthens because the system repeatedly observes meaningful change following the response.

Again, this is not moral failure. It is associative learning.

The nervous system continuously updates future prediction based on repeated outcomes. When a particular sequence repeatedly precedes reward or relief, the system increases readiness around that sequence. Anticipation becomes quicker. Salience becomes stronger. The pathway becomes easier to enter.

Internal pressure can intensify this process further.

Hunger may increase sensitivity toward reward-associated cues because appetite pressure increases relevance around intake and anticipated satisfaction. Fatigue may increase responsiveness toward convenience, stimulation, or familiarity because depleted systems assign greater value to expected restoration. Stress load may increase the salience of comfort-linked pathways because regulation becomes psychologically important under strain. Sleep debt, emotional exhaustion, glucose instability, and environmental availability can all make repeated loops easier to activate because the anticipated outcome feels more valuable under current conditions.

The stronger the internal pressure, the more motivational weight the predicted outcome may carry.

This interaction between reinforcement and internal state helps explain why some craving patterns feel far more automatic during periods of strain than during periods of stability. The repeated sequence already exists, but the current condition increases the relevance of the anticipated reward or relief. The loop becomes easier to activate because the expected outcome appears more meaningful.

Importantly, reinforcement operates gradually rather than all at once. Loops strengthen through accumulated repetition. The system becomes increasingly prepared around expected patterns because repeated exposure reduces uncertainty and increases predictive confidence.

A repeated sequence becomes easier to anticipate because the nervous system has practiced the pathway repeatedly.

This gradual strengthening can create the impression that cravings are becoming more "powerful" in a moral sense. But much of the change reflects efficiency rather than corruption. The system has learned what to expect. Familiar pathways become increasingly available because prediction becomes increasingly organized.

The emotional experience of craving may therefore begin earlier in the sequence over time. The cue activates anticipation more rapidly. The craving gains intensity more quickly. The expected outcome becomes psychologically available sooner. The pathway feels more immediate because the nervous system already recognizes the structure.

The response loop becomes partially self-maintaining because reinforcement strengthens future readiness. The system becomes increasingly prepared for what it repeatedly encounters. This preparation reduces the amount of uncertainty required before activation begins.

Importantly, understanding reinforcement structurally changes interpretation.

Without a systems frame, repeated cravings often appear personally condemning. The person sees repetition and concludes that something must be fundamentally wrong with them. But repeated activation patterns do not prove broken character. They demonstrate learned association strengthened through repetition.

A repeated craving pattern is not evidence that the person is weak. It is evidence that the system has practiced the sequence.

This reframing matters because moral interpretation often obscures the actual mechanism. The focus shifts toward self-judgment instead of toward understanding how cue recognition, prediction, repeated response, anticipated reward, and reinforcement interact across time. The pathway itself becomes invisible beneath shame-based interpretation.

A systems interpretation restores visibility to the process.

The craving becomes more understandable once reinforcement is recognized as pattern strengthening rather than character collapse. The loop grows faster, more automatic, and easier to activate because the nervous system has repeatedly linked cue, anticipation, response, and meaningful outcome.

The signal becomes more efficient because the sequence has become familiar.

Seen clearly, reinforcement is not proof that a person is broken or incapable of change. It is evidence that the system learned the pattern through repetition and now recognizes it quickly. The craving gains speed and automaticity because the nervous system has become increasingly prepared for a familiar predicted reward or relief pathway.

The loop becomes easier to activate not because the person has failed morally, but because the system has learned the sequence well enough to begin preparing for it before conscious deliberation fully unfolds.

Relief Encoding Mechanism

Pleasure is not the only outcome capable of reinforcing a craving loop. A response does not need to produce intense enjoyment in order to become behaviorally meaningful. In many cases, the response becomes reinforcing because it changes an uncomfortable state. The shift may be subtle or temporary, but the nervous system can still register the sequence as useful if pressure decreases, tension softens, discomfort quiets, or strain becomes easier to tolerate.

This distinction matters because craving is often interpreted too narrowly through pleasure alone. The signal appears reward-seeking, so the assumption becomes that the person is pursuing excess enjoyment, indulgence, or sensory gratification. But many craving loops strengthen not because the reward is overwhelmingly pleasurable, but because the response interrupts something unpleasant.

Relief can function as reward.

The system continuously evaluates changes in internal state. If discomfort is present and a particular response repeatedly reduces that discomfort, the reduction itself becomes behaviorally meaningful. The nervous system learns from state change. A response that softens strain, decreases agitation, interrupts boredom, reduces cognitive overload, or temporarily quiets emotional pressure may become increasingly associated with relief.

This is the Relief Encoding Mechanism.

The Relief Encoding Mechanism describes the process by which the system learns to repeat a craving-response pattern because the response reduces, interrupts, softens, or appears to reduce an uncomfortable internal state. The craving becomes reinforced because the response is linked not only with reward in the pleasurable sense, but with movement away from pressure.

This movement away from discomfort is often highly motivational.

Pleasure adds something desirable. Relief removes something uncomfortable.

The distinction is important because removal of discomfort can carry strong behavioral weight even when the resulting pleasure is modest. A response may not feel euphoric, dramatic, or intensely rewarding in a conventional sense. It may simply create less tension than the state that preceded it. But that reduction can still become reinforcing because the nervous system registers the change as meaningful.

A stressed system values decompression. A fatigued system values ease. An agitated system values interruption of strain. A bored system values stimulation. A restricted system values release from pressure. These shifts do not need to feel extraordinary in order to shape future prediction.

The response becomes associated with state change.

This association helps explain why some cravings feel emotionally urgent even when sensory pleasure itself is not especially intense. The anticipated outcome may involve reduction rather than addition. The system is not only moving toward enjoyment. It is moving away from discomfort.

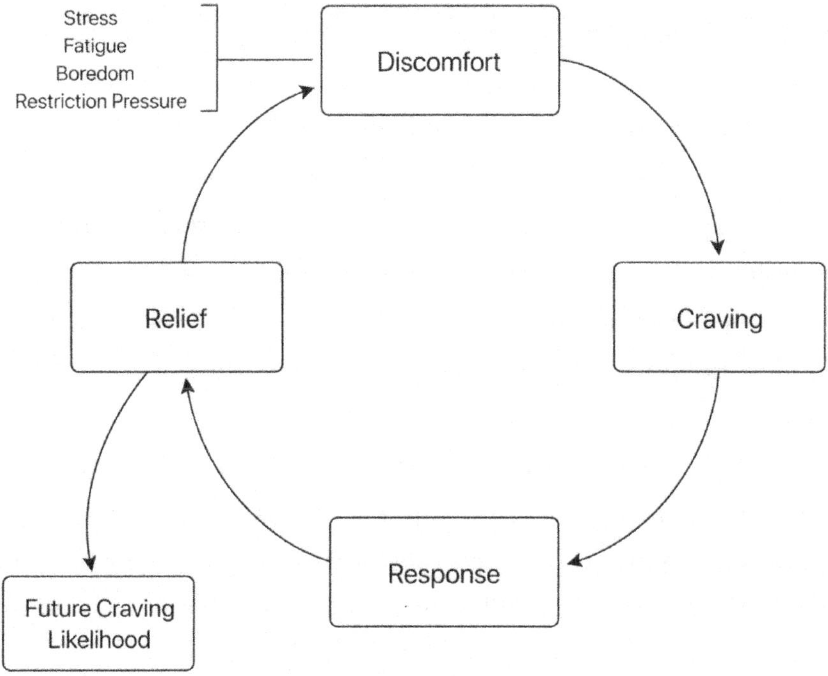

[Figure 9: Relief Reinforcement Loop]

The loop clarifies why discomfort reduction can strengthen future craving activation. A pressure state appears. The craving organizes around a predicted response. The response alters the state. Relief occurs, even if partially or temporarily. The nervous system learns that the sequence produced meaningful reduction in discomfort. Future pressure conditions begin activating the same pathway more quickly.

This learning process is normal rather than pathological.

Systems naturally move toward regulation and away from strain. Relief-seeking is not evidence of weak character, defective motivation, or emotional failure. Organisms continuously attempt to reduce unnecessary internal pressure. The significance of relief encoding is not that relief matters too much. The significance is that repeated pairings between discomfort and response can strengthen future activation patterns.

The system learns what appears to help.

This learning becomes especially important when pressure states occur repeatedly. If a specific response consistently softens tension, interrupts fatigue, reduces boredom, or provides temporary decompression, the nervous system begins assigning predictive value to that response. Future discomfort becomes increasingly likely to activate the associated craving pathway.

Stress often functions this way because stress narrows tolerance and increases the perceived value of rapid state change. Under sustained pressure, the system becomes increasingly attentive to anything associated with relief, interruption, familiarity, or decompression. A craving may therefore intensify not because the object itself is uniquely necessary, but because the anticipated reduction in strain feels psychologically important.

The craving becomes tied to expected relief from pressure.

A person under chronic stress may therefore experience strong anticipatory pull toward familiar sensory experiences, repeated routines, or comfort-associated responses because the nervous system has linked those patterns with temporary softening of overload. The reward is partly the interruption of strain itself.

This does not mean the response eliminates stress structurally. The relief may be partial, brief, inconsistent, or context-dependent. But temporary reduction in discomfort can still reinforce the pathway because the nervous system encodes meaningful change rather than permanent resolution.

The same logic applies to boredom.

Boredom is often underestimated because it appears emotionally neutral on the surface. But prolonged under-stimulation can create internal restlessness, cognitive discomfort, irritability, agitation, or a sense of unfinished activation. The system begins assigning value to experiences that interrupt monotony or increase salience.

A craving emerging during boredom may therefore function less as pursuit of pleasure and more as pursuit of interruption. The anticipated reward involves movement away from flatness, repetition, or under-stimulation. The response becomes meaningful because it changes the texture of the state itself.

Relief does not always mean comfort. Sometimes it means interruption.

This distinction helps explain why highly stimulating or sensory-intense experiences can become associated with craving under low-stimulation conditions. The nervous system learns that certain responses rapidly alter the felt environment. Future boredom increases readiness around those pathways because the anticipated state change has become behaviorally important.

Fatigue creates similar reinforcement pressures through a different route. A fatigued system often values convenience, ease, stimulation, familiarity, or rapid shifts in perceived capacity. Under exhaustion, responses associated with temporary activation or reduction in heaviness may gain salience because the current condition already feels difficult to sustain.

A craving under fatigue may therefore organize around expected relief from depletion rather than around sensory pleasure alone. The anticipated outcome may involve increased energy, interruption of heaviness, emotional softening, or reduction in the felt cost of continued effort.

Again, this does not require dramatic pleasure to become reinforcing. A slight improvement in tolerability can matter significantly when baseline strain is already elevated.

The nervous system learns from relative change, not only from intensity.

Restriction pressure introduces another important layer of relief encoding. When a person experiences prolonged suppression, rigid restraint, perceived scarcity, or sustained cognitive pressure surrounding reward-related behavior, the eventual release of that pressure can itself become reinforcing. The response may feel relieving partly because the state of suppression temporarily relaxes.

The significance here is not dietary morality. Restriction pressure can emerge in many forms whenever access, permission, or psychological flexibility becomes tightly constrained. The relief associated with release from restraint may therefore strengthen the craving-response pathway because the nervous system experiences reduction in tension.

The reinforcement may attach not only to the object itself, but to escape from suppression.

This helps explain why some craving experiences feel disproportionately intense after prolonged periods of rigidity or sustained internal control pressure. The anticipated outcome includes reduction of constraint. The response becomes psychologically meaningful because it alters the pressure state surrounding deprivation, tension, or restriction.

Emotional strain functions similarly without requiring clinical or diagnostic framing. Emotional discomfort can increase the salience of familiarity, warmth, predictability, comfort, sensory consistency, or interruption of distress. A response repeatedly associated with temporary emotional softening may become increasingly linked with relief prediction.

The craving therefore becomes organized around expected regulation.

The important distinction is that the system is not irrational for learning these associations. The nervous system continuously updates prediction according to repeated outcomes. If a certain response reliably softens emotional strain, reduces agitation, interrupts cognitive overload, or creates temporary relief from discomfort, the pathway becomes easier to activate later under similar conditions.

A craving can therefore become partially relief-seeking in structure.

This means the signal may not only communicate desire for food, taste, or pleasure. It may also carry expectation that a particular response will make the current state easier to tolerate. The anticipated outcome involves reduction of discomfort, not only addition of enjoyment.

Craving is often interpreted too narrowly because the relief layer remains hidden beneath the surface of the behavior. The person sees pursuit of reward and assumes pleasure is the entire explanation. But the nervous system may be orienting toward interruption of strain rather than toward excess enjoyment alone.

The expected state change becomes central.

This helps explain why some cravings feel especially persuasive under conditions of overload, emotional fatigue, cognitive exhaustion, loneliness, restlessness, or prolonged stress exposure. The anticipated response appears meaningful because it is associated with movement away from discomfort.

The stronger the pressure state, the more motivationally relevant relief may become.

Importantly, relief encoding does not require the relief to be complete or even fully accurate. The response may only partially soften discomfort. The improvement may be temporary. The anticipated relief may exceed the actual effect. But repeated pairings between discomfort and even modest reduction in strain can still strengthen future prediction.

The system learns that the sequence changes the state.

This predictive learning can become highly efficient over time. Internal discomfort begins activating anticipation rapidly because the nervous system already recognizes the familiar pattern. Stress predicts decompression. Fatigue predicts stimulation or convenience. Restriction predicts release. Boredom predicts interruption. Emotional strain predicts comfort or familiarity.

The craving emerges because the system expects movement away from discomfort.

A response that repeatedly reduces pressure becomes easier to anticipate and easier to pursue.

Again, none of this requires moral interpretation. Relief-seeking is not inherently excessive or irrational. Regulation is a basic feature of living systems. The issue is not that discomfort reduction matters. The issue is that repeated relief pairing teaches the nervous system which pathways appear useful under strain.

This learning process can make future cravings feel increasingly automatic because the pressure state itself becomes part of the cue structure. Stress, fatigue, boredom, agitation, restriction, loneliness, cognitive overload, or emotional strain begin functioning as predictive conditions that activate expected relief.

The internal state becomes a learned activation signal.

This also explains why some cravings feel less connected to sensory enjoyment than to emotional urgency or state intolerance. The craving may carry strong motivational pull because the anticipated outcome involves relief from pressure rather than pursuit of pleasure alone.

A person may therefore experience intense wanting even when the eventual pleasure is moderate. The behavioral force belongs partly to expected reduction in discomfort. The nervous system prioritizes the possibility of relief because the current condition already feels strained.

The more consistently a response appears to soften pressure, the more strongly the association may become encoded.

Relief teaches the system through contrast.

The contrast between discomfort and temporary reduction creates learning significance. The nervous system notices that the state changed. Future prediction becomes organized around repeating the sequence under similar conditions.

Understanding relief encoding changes how repeated craving loops are interpreted. Without a systems frame, relief-seeking behavior is often moralized as weakness, lack of discipline, emotional instability, or excessive dependence on reward. But much of the reinforcement may be occurring because the nervous system has repeatedly linked a certain response with reduction of strain.

The repeated loop reflects learned association, not broken character.

This distinction restores structural clarity. The craving becomes understandable as prediction organized around anticipated relief. The system is not merely seeking pleasure for its own sake. Often it is attempting to alter an uncomfortable internal condition that has become difficult to sustain.

Seen clearly, a craving may be carrying the prediction that a familiar response will reduce tension, soften fatigue, interrupt boredom, quiet agitation, release restriction pressure, or make emotional strain more tolerable. The signal becomes reinforced because the nervous system has learned that the sequence appears to help change the state.

Future discomfort therefore activates the pathway more quickly.

The craving loop gains efficiency because the system has learned the association between pressure and expected relief. The signal becomes more understandable once reinforcement is recognized not as evidence of weak character, but as the nervous system repeatedly preparing for a familiar form of discomfort reduction.

Memory Reactivation Mechanism

Cravings often feel immediate because memory has already organized the signal before conscious awareness fully catches up. A person encounters a cue, transition, environment, emotional state, sensory detail, or familiar routine, and the craving appears suddenly, almost as though it emerged spontaneously in the present moment. But many cravings are not constructed entirely from present conditions. They are reactivated from stored associations built through prior experience.

The system does not respond only to what is happening now. It also responds to what similar conditions have meant before.

A familiar cue may therefore reactivate a prior reward pattern long before the person consciously narrates the process. The craving feels current, but the pathway itself may already exist in stored form. Previous experiences involving reward, relief, comfort, stimulation, decompression, familiarity, or emotional softening remain behaviorally relevant because the nervous system retains predictive associations between context and expected outcome.

This is the Memory Reactivation Mechanism.

The Memory Reactivation Mechanism describes the process by which stored associations between prior reward, emotional state, cue, context, response, and relief are reactivated when similar internal or external conditions appear, making craving feel familiar, specific, and quickly available. The craving gains force because the system retrieves a previously learned pattern and restores its predictive structure into the present moment.

Memory therefore functions as active prediction infrastructure rather than passive archival storage.

A craving may feel immediate because the pathway was already prepared.

This distinction changes how craving intensity is interpreted. The signal is not necessarily being built from scratch each time. In many cases, the nervous system is retrieving an already organized pattern involving expected reward, emotional tone, sensory familiarity, contextual association, and anticipated state change. The craving feels convincing partly because the pathway has been experienced before.

The system remembers outcomes that appeared meaningful.

A prior response associated with pleasure, comfort, decompression, stimulation, relief, regulation, familiarity, emotional softening, or interruption of strain may remain behaviorally available long after the original experience ends. Future cues can reactivate that stored association because memory preserves predictive relevance across time.

Craving therefore becomes partly a retrieval process.

A present cue activates remembered reward. Remembered reward increases expected outcome salience. Increased expectation strengthens craving availability. The nervous system begins preparing for the familiar sequence because memory reconnects cue, anticipation, response, and predicted effect.

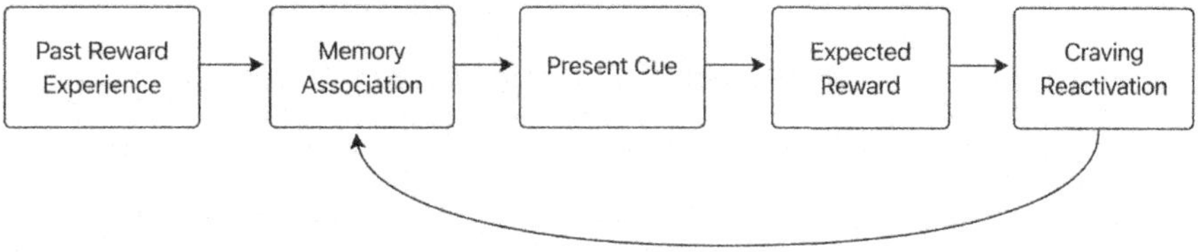

[Figure 10: Memory Reactivation Pathway]

The pathway matters because it shows that memory does not merely recall prior experiences in a passive narrative sense. Memory restores the predictive structure surrounding them. The present cue activates stored association. The stored association reactivates expected reward. Expected reward strengthens motivational pull. The craving becomes available because the nervous system recognizes a familiar pathway and begins orienting toward it again.

Memory does not simply recall the reward. It restores the pathway toward it.

This restoration process can happen rapidly because familiarity reduces uncertainty. A previously learned pattern requires less information for activation than a novel one. The system already recognizes the sequence. A relatively small cue can therefore reactivate a much larger network of association involving sensory expectation, emotional tone, anticipated relief, contextual familiarity, and behavioral readiness.

This helps explain why cravings often feel surprisingly specific. The remembered pathway itself was specific.

The system may not only remember a general category of reward. It may preserve texture, temperature, smell, timing, environment, emotional atmosphere, convenience, sensory intensity, social context, or anticipated effect. A craving therefore gains direction because the stored association already contains organized detail.

Sensory memory becomes especially important here because many reward experiences are encoded through repeated sensory patterns. Texture, sweetness, saltiness, warmth, crunch, creaminess, temperature contrast, speed of access, or familiar combinations of sensation can remain strongly linked to anticipated reward or relief long after the original experience occurred.

The nervous system remembers how the experience felt.

A particular flavor profile may become associated with decompression after stress. A familiar texture may become linked with comfort or emotional softening. A specific sensory intensity may become associated with stimulation during boredom or fatigue. The craving becomes targeted because memory preserved the details surrounding the expected outcome.

This specificity does not indicate biological necessity. It reflects organized prediction.

The more consistently certain sensory experiences were linked with meaningful state change, the easier those associations become to retrieve later. A familiar sensory cue can therefore reactivate expectation quickly because the nervous system already recognizes its prior significance.

Emotional tone also becomes part of memory architecture.

Memory is not merely factual storage. The nervous system often preserves the emotional atmosphere surrounding prior reward experiences. Relief, comfort, decompression, celebration, stimulation, safety, familiarity, distraction, interruption of loneliness, reduction of cognitive overload, or temporary quieting of tension can all become integrated into the remembered pattern.

The emotional condition becomes linked with the expected outcome.

A craving may therefore reactivate not only a sensory target, but an anticipated emotional shift associated with prior experiences. The system remembers that the sequence previously altered the state in a meaningful way. The anticipated emotional effect becomes behaviorally relevant again when similar conditions appear.

This process does not require dramatic psychological interpretation. Emotional association is a normal feature of learning systems. Experiences occurring during emotionally meaningful states are often encoded with stronger predictive significance because the nervous system treats emotionally relevant information as behaviorally important.

A remembered reward therefore carries more than taste. It often carries atmosphere.

This helps explain why cravings can emerge strongly during familiar emotional conditions even when physical hunger remains relatively stable. Stress, loneliness, fatigue, boredom, agitation, emotional strain, cognitive overload, or restlessness may reactivate stored patterns because the internal state resembles conditions previously associated with meaningful relief or reward.

The system recognizes emotional similarity.

Context-linked memory strengthens this process further because the nervous system stores experiences relationally rather than in isolation. The remembered pattern often includes environmental conditions surrounding the prior reward experience. Times of day, rooms, routes, seasons, screens, stores, sounds, lighting conditions, social settings, routines, and transition periods may all become linked with expected outcomes.

The craving therefore does not emerge independently from context. It emerges through contextual retrieval.

A driving route associated with repeated reward experiences may reactivate anticipation before conscious reflection occurs. A familiar evening transition may restore expected decompression. A particular room, lighting pattern, or entertainment environment may reactivate comfort-associated prediction because memory preserved the surrounding structure alongside the reward itself.

The system remembers sequences, not isolated objects.

This is one reason cravings can feel highly situational. The environment helps restore the predictive architecture surrounding prior reward experiences. The cue becomes meaningful because memory already linked it with anticipated state change.

Importantly, memory reactivation does not require deliberate remembering. A person does not need to consciously revisit a prior experience in narrative detail for the associated pathway to become active. The nervous system can retrieve predictive relevance automatically when familiar conditions appear. The craving may therefore feel sudden because the stored pattern became active before conscious awareness organized the experience verbally.

The system retrieves association faster than explanation.

This distinction matters because cravings are often interpreted as spontaneous impulses disconnected from prior learning. In reality, much of the activation may occur beneath deliberate reflection. The person notices the craving after the predictive pathway has already begun reorganizing attention, expectation, and salience around the anticipated outcome.

The activation feels immediate because memory compresses the sequence.

A relatively small cue can retrieve a much larger stored architecture involving sensory expectation, emotional tone, anticipated relief, contextual familiarity, and response readiness. The nervous system already understands the pathway, so less activation is required to bring the craving forward.

Familiar loops reactivate quickly because they have already been practiced.

A pathway repeatedly associated with meaningful reward or relief becomes increasingly efficient over time. Familiarity lowers activation threshold because the system recognizes the sequence rapidly. A small amount of matching information becomes enough to retrieve a larger predictive structure.

The craving therefore feels convincing partly because the expected outcome feels familiar.

Familiarity increases trust in prediction.

A previously experienced response carries psychological credibility because the nervous system has already linked it with meaningful state change. Even if the actual outcome later proves partial, temporary, inconsistent, or mixed, the familiarity of the pathway itself can strengthen anticipation in advance.

The expected effect feels believable because it has been experienced before.

This helps explain why cravings can remain persuasive even after imperfect outcomes. The nervous system stores prior meaningful associations and retrieves them quickly when matching conditions appear. Prediction is organized around remembered significance rather than around objective certainty.

Memory therefore functions as reinforcement architecture.

It preserves the structure of prior loops: cue, anticipation, response, reward, relief, emotional tone, sensory profile, context, and expected state change. The architecture remains behaviorally available after the original experience ends. Future activation becomes faster because the system no longer needs to construct the sequence from the beginning.

The pathway already exists in stored form.

This architectural function is critical because it allows craving to develop speed and efficiency across repeated experiences. The nervous system learns not only isolated rewards, but entire predictive sequences linking conditions with outcomes. The more often the sequence repeats, the more rapidly the architecture can be reactivated later.

Memory stores prediction pathways, not merely events.

This distinction keeps the chapter inside the systems frame rather than drifting into nostalgic or autobiographical interpretation. The issue is not that people emotionally dwell on past rewards in a reflective sense. The issue is that prior reward experiences remain structurally active through stored association. The nervous system continues using past experience to organize future prediction.

Memory can preserve both the object and the surrounding state.

The system may remember the food, but also the room, the timing, the social atmosphere, the emotional pressure that preceded the response, the relief that followed, the sensory intensity, the transition surrounding the experience, and the familiarity of the sequence itself. The craving returns with recognizable direction because the stored architecture contains much more than the object alone.

This helps explain why cravings often feel emotionally layered even before the response occurs. The pathway already includes remembered atmosphere and anticipated state change. The craving carries predictive familiarity because memory preserved the relational structure surrounding the prior experience.

Internal state can strengthen memory reactivation significantly. Stress, fatigue, emotional strain, boredom, restriction pressure, loneliness, cognitive overload, glucose instability, sleep debt, and environmental availability can all increase the salience of stored reward pathways because the current condition resembles states previously associated with meaningful relief or regulation.

The stronger the resemblance, the easier retrieval may become.

A fatigued state may reactivate convenience-associated prediction quickly because the system remembers prior reduction in effort or heaviness. Emotional strain may reactivate comfort-linked pathways because the nervous system previously associated those responses with temporary softening of pressure. Stress may reactivate decompression-associated sequences because memory preserved the anticipated reduction in overload.

Again, this does not make the craving irrational or morally suspect. The nervous system is functioning predictively. It retrieves pathways that previously appeared meaningful under similar conditions.

Memory architecture increases efficiency through familiarity.

This familiarity can make craving feel deeply convincing because the anticipated outcome already carries stored experiential weight. The nervous system does not treat the prediction as abstract possibility. It recognizes the pathway as previously meaningful and therefore worthy of renewed attention.

A familiar prediction feels more real than an unfamiliar one.

This helps explain why some cravings appear to arrive with emotional certainty even before the anticipated reward occurs. The certainty belongs partly to retrieval efficiency. The pathway already exists in organized form. Memory restored the structure rapidly.

Importantly, this process can occur without strong hunger or broad biological depletion. The nervous system may reactivate a stored reward pathway because the cue and context resemble prior meaningful experiences, even when energy need itself remains relatively stable.

The craving becomes active because prediction became active.

This distinction prevents craving from being interpreted only through physical need. The signal may emerge from remembered association rather than from immediate depletion. The system recognizes familiar conditions and restores the expected sequence into present awareness.

Seen clearly, memory reactivation makes craving more understandable and less mysterious. The craving is not appearing from nowhere. The nervous system encountered a familiar cue, retrieved a stored association, restored expected reward, and began preparing for a previously learned response.

The signal becomes readable once memory is understood as reinforcement architecture rather than passive recall.

The craving feels familiar because the pathway is familiar. The specificity exists because the stored pattern was specific. The emotional tone returns because the association preserved emotional context alongside reward and relief. The speed of activation increases because memory compresses the predictive sequence into efficient retrieval.

A repeated craving therefore reflects stored learning becoming active again.

The system recognizes conditions resembling prior meaningful experiences and rapidly restores the associated pathway toward anticipated reward, relief, comfort, stimulation, familiarity, or regulation. The craving becomes understandable once it is interpreted not as sudden moral failure, but as memory reactivating a learned reinforcement structure already embedded within the system.

Appetite Pressure Mechanism

Craving intensity often changes when the system is already under appetite pressure. A reward signal that might remain relatively quiet under stable conditions can become more urgent, more specific, and more behaviorally persuasive when hunger, delayed intake, unstable satiety, underfeeding, restriction pressure, or perceived scarcity are present. The craving itself may still be organized around reward prediction, sensory specificity, familiarity, or anticipated relief, but the surrounding physiological pressure gives the signal additional force.

This distinction matters because appetite pressure and craving are often treated as identical experiences. They overlap frequently, but they are not the same process. Appetite pressure is broader. It reflects accumulated intake relevance, unresolved hunger, unstable satisfaction, delayed restoration, or increased motivational importance surrounding food and reward. Craving is narrower. It tends to organize around a particular target, expected outcome, sensory profile, or learned association.

The two systems interact continuously.

Hunger may provide pressure while craving supplies direction.

This interaction helps explain why cravings often become dramatically more persuasive under conditions of depletion, instability, or perceived restriction. The specific target may already exist as a learned reward pathway, but appetite pressure amplifies its motivational pull. The signal gains intensity because the system is already operating under increased food relevance.

This is the Appetite Pressure Mechanism.

The Appetite Pressure Mechanism describes the process by which accumulated hunger, unstable satiety, perceived scarcity, restriction pressure, or delayed intake increases the force of reward signals and makes cravings feel more urgent, specific, and behaviorally compelling. Appetite pressure does not create every craving, but it increases the salience and motivational weight of existing reward pathways.

The system becomes more responsive to anticipated reward when broader intake pressure rises.

A familiar sensory cue may therefore feel stronger under conditions of hunger than under conditions of stability. A remembered reward may appear more persuasive when satiety feels incomplete or uncertain. A previously mild craving may become emotionally urgent because broad appetite pressure is increasing the value assigned to expected intake, relief, comfort, stimulation, or restoration.

The craving gains volume because the surrounding system state has changed.

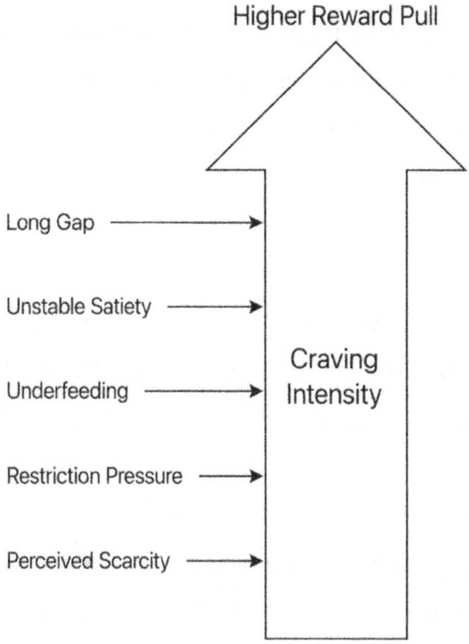

[Figure 11: Appetite Pressure Amplifier]

The amplifier model is important because it clarifies that appetite pressure acts on existing reward signals rather than replacing them. A specific craving may still be organized around texture, familiarity, anticipated relief, emotional association, convenience, sensory intensity, or remembered reward. Appetite pressure increases the signal's force by increasing the overall motivational relevance of intake and restoration.

Under stable conditions, a reward cue may remain relatively mild because the system is not assigning high urgency to intake-related possibilities. Under pressure, the same cue may feel significantly more persuasive because broad intake relevance has increased.

Appetite pressure therefore functions as a force multiplier.

Underfeeding illustrates this clearly because low intake relative to demand increases the motivational significance of reward-related cues. The nervous system becomes increasingly attentive to opportunities associated with intake, restoration, or expected relief from deprivation. This does not require dramatic starvation conditions. Even moderate reductions in perceived availability, unresolved hunger, or prolonged insufficiency can increase reward salience.

The system becomes more sensitive when restoration feels incomplete.

A cue associated with comfort, sensory intensity, familiarity, convenience, or rapid intake may therefore become more psychologically important under conditions of underfeeding because the nervous system is already prioritizing intake relevance broadly. The specific craving gains additional pull because the surrounding metabolic environment has elevated the importance of food-related signals.

Long gaps can create similar amplification because delayed intake extends the period during which appetite pressure accumulates. The nervous system continues tracking unresolved food relevance across time. As the gap lengthens, reward-associated signals may become increasingly salient because the system is operating under rising motivational pressure surrounding intake and restoration.

Again, the important distinction is that appetite pressure is not identical to craving itself. A person may experience broad hunger without strong specificity. But when a specific reward pathway becomes activated during periods of elevated appetite pressure, the craving often feels more urgent and behaviorally persuasive.

The pressure amplifies the pathway already present.

This amplification can make cravings feel biologically necessary even when the craving's specificity remains largely organized around learned reward prediction rather than pure energy need. A person may therefore experience intense certainty surrounding a highly specific target because broad appetite pressure is increasing the force of an already familiar reward association.

The signal feels essential because multiple layers are converging simultaneously.

Unstable satiety contributes to this process differently. Satiety instability does not necessarily mean complete absence of intake. A person may have eaten and still experience persistent return of food relevance because the system does not fully settle into stable resolution. Appetite remains partially active. Food-related attention continues returning. Reward-associated cues remain highly available because the broader motivational state surrounding intake never fully quiets.

The result can be heightened sensitivity to specific reward signals.

When satiety remains unstable, the nervous system continues assigning importance to intake-related possibilities. Craving pathways therefore encounter less resistance from broader physiological settling. The reward signal becomes easier to activate because the system is already maintaining elevated food relevance.

This can create situations where a person feels confused about why craving persists despite recent intake. But the issue may not be simple absence of food. The issue may involve unresolved appetite pressure interacting with learned reward pathways, sensory expectation, or anticipated relief.

Satiety instability keeps the system partially open to reward activation.

Restriction pressure introduces another powerful amplifier because perceived scarcity changes motivational valuation. When access feels uncertain, constrained, forbidden, delayed, tightly controlled, or psychologically restricted, the restricted object often gains additional salience. The nervous system increases attention toward what appears limited because scarcity increases perceived importance.

Restriction pressure therefore changes reward intensity.

This does not require moral interpretation of restraint itself. The systems question is not whether all restriction is inherently harmful or irrational. The systems question is how perceived scarcity alters motivational organization surrounding reward-related signals.

When access feels constrained, anticipated release from restriction can itself become reinforcing.

The craving may therefore intensify not only because the object is rewarding, but because the object becomes associated with restoration of access, interruption of deprivation, or reduction of tension surrounding limitation. The restricted target gains additional psychological weight because scarcity increases perceived value.

Perceived scarcity magnifies salience.

This helps explain why specific cravings can become especially intense during periods of rigid control, prolonged suppression, unresolved deprivation, or sustained cognitive focus on limitation. The nervous system begins assigning greater importance to the anticipated reward because the broader environment communicates reduced availability.

The less available something feels, the more behaviorally important it may become.

Importantly, this amplification process is not purely sensory. Appetite pressure alters prediction itself. Under conditions of deprivation or instability, the expected value of reward rises because restoration appears increasingly meaningful. The anticipated outcome gains emotional and motivational weight before the response occurs.

Deprivation changes the emotional size of reward.

A familiar comfort-associated experience may therefore feel unusually important during periods of hunger, fatigue, restriction pressure, or unresolved appetite because the nervous system predicts stronger restoration value under strained conditions. The craving becomes more persuasive because the expected state change feels more necessary.

Convenience can also gain salience under appetite pressure because rapid access to intake becomes increasingly behaviorally relevant when restoration feels delayed or uncertain. The system assigns value not only to the reward itself, but to speed of resolution. Familiarity, immediacy, sensory intensity, and predictability may all become more compelling because appetite pressure increases the urgency surrounding restoration.

The signal narrows around what appears quickly resolving.

This narrowing helps explain why cravings under appetite pressure often become highly specific. The nervous system is not merely searching abstractly for food. It is organizing around targets associated with efficient anticipated restoration, familiar reward, sensory certainty, or expected relief.

The craving gains force because the system predicts meaningful reduction in pressure.

Memory and cue association become especially important under these conditions because appetite pressure increases responsiveness to already established reward pathways. A familiar cue that might feel manageable under stable conditions can become highly persuasive when broad hunger or perceived scarcity is elevated. The cue activates remembered reward while appetite pressure amplifies the motivational relevance of that prediction.

Stored associations gain additional leverage under strain.

A familiar sensory memory may therefore feel unusually convincing during periods of underfeeding or unresolved hunger because the system already recognizes the pathway as meaningful and now assigns increased urgency to restoration. Appetite pressure and memory reactivation reinforce one another.

Cue association functions similarly. Environmental signals linked with prior reward become more salient when the nervous system is already operating under elevated intake relevance. A familiar time of day, social setting, screen environment, emotional state, or transition period may activate craving more strongly because appetite pressure increases sensitivity to reward-associated cues.

The cue becomes louder when the system is already listening for restoration.

Importantly, appetite pressure does not erase the distinction between hunger and craving. The broader intake pressure may increase intensity, but the craving's specificity still often reflects prediction, learned association, sensory familiarity, anticipated relief, emotional memory, or reinforcement history.

This distinction prevents oversimplification.

A person experiencing strong appetite pressure may still develop highly targeted cravings because the broad motivational state amplifies specific learned reward pathways rather than replacing them. The craving feels biologically urgent because broad hunger and narrow reward prediction have merged into a single persuasive signal.

The pressure belongs to hunger. The direction belongs to prediction.

This interaction can make cravings feel deeply convincing because the nervous system is combining broad restoration relevance with specific anticipated reward. The expected outcome appears behaviorally important on multiple levels simultaneously. Hunger increases urgency while memory, cue association, familiarity, and anticipated relief provide precision.

The resulting signal can feel disproportionately powerful relative to the actual object itself because the craving now carries amplified motivational weight from the surrounding metabolic state.

Again, none of this requires moral interpretation. Appetite pressure is not evidence of failed discipline. Underfeeding, prolonged gaps, unstable satiety, restriction pressure, and perceived scarcity naturally alter motivational salience surrounding intake-related signals. The nervous system responds adaptively to changing conditions by increasing the importance assigned to restoration-related opportunities.

The system prioritizes what appears relevant under current conditions.

This also explains why cravings can fluctuate dramatically depending on system state even when external conditions remain similar. The same cue may feel relatively mild under stable conditions and highly compelling under elevated appetite pressure because the surrounding motivational environment changed.

The craving itself did not necessarily become fundamentally different. The amplifier changed.

Appetite pressure therefore helps explain why certain reward signals become unusually emotionally charged during periods of deprivation, instability, or unresolved intake relevance. The nervous system assigns greater urgency to anticipated restoration because broad physiological pressure increases the value of reward-associated pathways.

A craving intensified by appetite pressure is not proof of weak character. It is evidence that the system is operating under increased motivational relevance surrounding intake, restoration, and expected relief.

Seen clearly, appetite pressure makes craving more understandable rather than more morally loaded. The craving becomes amplified because the nervous system is combining broad hunger-related pressure with specific learned reward prediction. Underfeeding, long gaps, unstable satiety, restriction pressure, and perceived scarcity increase the force of reward signals by increasing the perceived importance of restoration itself.

The signal feels stronger because the system state gives it more force.

Glucose Urgency Mechanism

Some cravings become urgent not merely because reward is expected, but because the system senses instability in fuel availability. A reward signal that might remain interpretable and manageable under stable conditions can become sharper, faster, and more behaviorally persuasive when energy feels unstable, inconsistent, or difficult to sustain. The craving changes because the surrounding metabolic environment changes. Perceived instability increases the value of rapid state change.

This distinction matters because urgency is often interpreted morally rather than structurally. A sudden, intense craving may appear excessive, irrational, or personally alarming because of how immediate the signal feels. But in many cases, the intensity reflects the nervous system assigning priority to rapid restoration under conditions of perceived fuel instability.

The system becomes more sensitive when availability feels uncertain.

This is the Glucose Urgency Mechanism.

The Glucose Urgency Mechanism describes the process by which perceived fuel instability, glucose variability, energy dips, or crash-like states increase the urgency of reward signals by making rapid state change feel more valuable. The craving gains force because the nervous system interprets quick restoration as increasingly important when energy availability feels unstable.

Under stable conditions, a reward cue may remain relatively moderate in intensity because the surrounding system state feels adequately supported. The nervous system can interpret the signal without assigning immediate priority to it. But when energy feels unstable, the same cue can become highly persuasive because the expected reward appears capable of changing the current state quickly.

Instability changes the value of speed.

This helps explain why certain cravings feel qualitatively different during periods of shakiness, fog, heaviness, irritability, fatigue, restlessness, or perceived crashing than they do under steadier conditions. The reward signal becomes fused with urgency because the system is no longer evaluating reward in a neutral context. It is evaluating reward while operating under perceived instability.

The craving becomes tied to rapid correction.

Glucose movement is part of a larger coordinated regulation system involving intake, storage, release, utilization, hormonal signaling, stress activation, activity demand, recovery capacity, and ongoing metabolic adjustment. The purpose of this chapter is not to reteach that broader system in detail. The important point here is that unstable fuel availability changes motivational salience.

When the system senses instability, rapid reward becomes more behaviorally important.

The nervous system continuously monitors conditions related to usable energy and restoration. When energy feels stable, the urgency surrounding intake often decreases. But when availability appears inconsistent, unreliable, rapidly dropping, or difficult to maintain, the system increases attentional priority around signals associated with fast state change.

A craving under these conditions may not only be about pleasure. It may involve expected restoration of clarity, steadiness, alertness, emotional tolerance, reduced heaviness, improved capacity, interruption of shakiness, or escape from crash-like discomfort.

The anticipated outcome becomes corrective in emotional tone.

This distinction is important because it changes how the craving feels subjectively. The signal often becomes more immediate and more persuasive because the nervous system is organizing around perceived restoration rather than around optional enjoyment alone. The expected reward appears behaviorally urgent because the current condition feels unstable.

A stable system can evaluate reward. An unstable system may prioritize it.

Energy dips illustrate this process clearly. When perceived fuel availability drops, the nervous system often becomes more responsive to signals associated with quick restoration. The craving narrows around experiences linked with rapid state change because speed itself acquires motivational value.

The person may not consciously analyze the sequence in metabolic terms. The experience simply feels urgent. A specific reward becomes emotionally important because the system predicts that the response may rapidly alter the current state.

Fog, shakiness, heaviness, irritability, reduced tolerance, restlessness, or feelings of crashing can all intensify this urgency because unstable conditions increase the perceived value of rapid intake or rapid relief. The craving becomes sharper because the nervous system is attempting to move toward stabilization.

The faster the expected correction, the stronger the pull may become.

This does not mean the system is perfectly precise in predicting what will fully restore stability. Cravings are still shaped by memory, reinforcement history, cue association, sensory familiarity, and anticipated reward. But under conditions of perceived instability, the motivational force surrounding fast-acting or familiar reward pathways often increases because the nervous system is prioritizing immediacy.

Rapid reward feels emotionally efficient under unstable conditions.

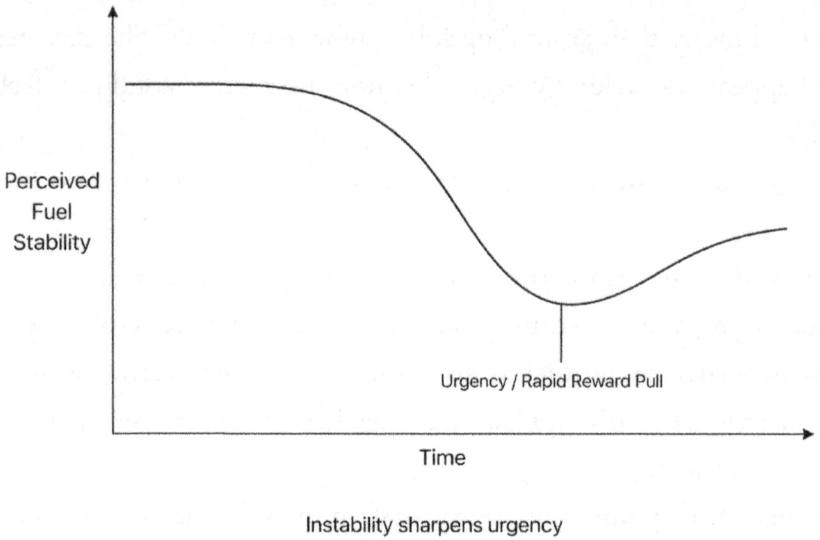

[Figure 12: Glucose Urgency Pattern]

The graph matters because it illustrates that urgency often rises at the point where perceived stability drops. The craving becomes more behaviorally compelling not necessarily because the reward itself changed, but because the surrounding system state changed. The dip increases the value assigned to rapid restoration.

This is one reason crash-like states can make cravings feel unusually authoritative. The nervous system narrows attention around what appears capable of changing the state quickly. The signal acquires emotional intensity because stabilization feels immediately relevant.

The craving begins to feel less like preference and more like necessity.

Importantly, this does not mean every urgent craving reflects severe physiological crisis or medical dysfunction. The chapter is describing recognizable states of perceived instability rather than diagnosing disease. Experiences such as shakiness, heaviness, fog, irritability, reduced patience, cognitive dullness, urgency, restlessness, or lowered frustration tolerance can all increase motivational responsiveness to rapid reward cues without requiring pathological framing.

The nervous system responds to perceived instability by increasing attentional priority around restoration-related possibilities.

This process becomes especially powerful when rapid reward pathways are already familiar. A remembered sensory experience associated with quick energy, fast relief, stimulation, or interruption of heaviness becomes more persuasive because the system already recognizes the pathway as potentially useful under unstable conditions.

Memory amplifies urgency when restoration feels uncertain.

A familiar fast-relief signal therefore gains additional force during periods of perceived instability because the nervous system already associates the pathway with meaningful state change. The craving becomes more convincing because prediction and urgency are operating simultaneously.

The system remembers what previously felt rapidly restoring.

This helps explain why cravings during energy dips often become highly specific. The nervous system is not merely searching abstractly for intake. It narrows around targets associated with immediacy, familiarity, sensory certainty, rapid accessibility, or previously experienced restoration.

Specificity increases because urgency prefers recognizable pathways.

Sweetness, convenience, intensity, rapid access, familiar sensory patterns, and predictability may all become more salient because unstable conditions increase the value of fast anticipated change. Again, this does not mean the craving is biologically exact or morally authoritative. It means the system is assigning urgency to pathways associated with rapid state alteration.

The craving feels convincing because the predicted outcome appears immediately relevant.

This is also why glucose-related urgency can sometimes feel emotionally disproportionate relative to the actual object involved. The emotional force belongs partly to the instability state itself. The reward cue becomes amplified because the nervous system is attempting to restore steadiness quickly.

Urgency compresses interpretation.

Under stable conditions, a person may recognize a craving as optional, contextual, or mild. Under unstable conditions, the same craving may feel urgent, emotionally loaded, or difficult to delay because the nervous system is assigning higher priority to rapid state change.

The signal gains force because tolerance narrows under instability.

Crash-like states intensify this further because they often involve more than physical sensation alone. Reduced patience, emotional irritability, mental fog, heaviness, shakiness, frustration sensitivity, and lowered cognitive flexibility can all make rapid restoration feel increasingly important. The craving becomes psychologically amplified because the current condition feels increasingly difficult to sustain.

The system seeks stabilization through speed.

This helps explain why convenience and immediacy become especially behaviorally relevant during periods of perceived fuel instability. The nervous system begins favoring pathways associated with fast correction because the emotional value of waiting, uncertainty, or delayed restoration decreases under strain.

Again, this does not require moral interpretation. The urgency is not evidence of weak discipline or personal failure. The nervous system naturally increases motivational priority around rapid restoration when conditions feel unstable.

A pressured system values immediacy.

This interaction becomes even stronger when appetite pressure is already elevated. Hunger, delayed intake, unstable satiety, restriction pressure, or perceived scarcity can combine with glucose variability to amplify reward urgency further. Broad appetite pressure increases food relevance while instability increases the value of rapid correction.

The craving gains both pressure and speed.

Under these conditions, familiar reward pathways can become extremely persuasive because multiple amplification systems are converging simultaneously. Hunger increases motivational relevance. Instability increases urgency. Memory supplies familiar restoration patterns. Cue association increases salience. Anticipated relief strengthens emotional pull.

The resulting craving may feel unusually commanding because several layers of prediction and pressure are operating together.

Importantly, glucose urgency does not eliminate the distinction between craving and biological need. A craving under unstable conditions may still organize around highly specific sensory targets, familiar reward pathways, emotional associations, or anticipated relief patterns. The urgency often reflects instability amplifying prediction rather than purely objective physiological necessity.

The system may be broadly seeking restoration while the craving narrows around a specific remembered pathway.

This distinction keeps the chapter inside the broader systems frame. Blood sugar regulation itself involves coordinated glucose movement, insulin signaling, liver release, activity demand, stress load, recovery state, sleep quality, and metabolic flexibility. Those layers matter because instability does not arise from one isolated variable. But the focus here is narrower: unstable availability sharpens reward urgency.

The nervous system assigns more value to rapid change when steadiness feels threatened.

This is one reason cravings can intensify dramatically during periods of exhaustion, prolonged stress, irregular intake, insufficient recovery, sleep disruption, emotional strain, or fluctuating energy availability. The system becomes increasingly attentive to anything associated with rapid perceived stabilization.

The craving becomes emotionally immediate because restoration feels behaviorally urgent.

Importantly, this process can occur even when the actual outcome later proves partial, temporary, or mixed. Anticipated restoration often feels highly convincing before the response occurs because the nervous system is organizing around expected relief from instability. The emotional force belongs partly to the prediction of rapid correction.

A remembered fast-relief pathway can therefore remain highly persuasive even when previous outcomes were imperfect because the nervous system continues prioritizing the possibility of quick stabilization under unstable conditions.

The signal says: change this state quickly.

Seen clearly, glucose urgency makes craving more understandable and less morally confusing. The craving becomes amplified because perceived fuel instability increases the emotional importance of rapid restoration. Energy dips, shakiness, fog, irritability, heaviness, crash-like states, or fluctuating availability all increase the salience of pathways associated with fast state change.

The system narrows around what appears rapidly restoring because instability increases the value of immediacy.

A craving intensified by unstable fuel conditions is therefore not proof of weak discipline or failed self-control. It is a reward signal amplified by the nervous system's attempt to move toward steadiness under conditions of perceived instability. The urgency belongs to the system's search for rapid restoration, not to moral failure.

Fatigue Reactivity Mechanism

Fatigue changes the way cravings are experienced because fatigue changes available capacity. A reward signal that might remain manageable, interpretable, or psychologically distant under rested conditions can feel more immediate, more persuasive, and more difficult to hold at distance under recovery debt. The craving itself may not be fundamentally different in structure, but the system encountering the craving has changed. Tolerance narrows. Reflective distance decreases. Effort becomes more expensive. The nervous system begins assigning greater value to what appears fast, familiar, and low-friction.

This distinction matters because cravings under fatigue are often interpreted morally rather than structurally. A person may experience stronger reward pull during periods of exhaustion and conclude that discipline has weakened or self-control has failed. But fatigue changes the operating conditions of the system itself. The same craving encountered under different capacity states does not carry the same psychological cost.

Fatigue alters the distance between signal and response.

This is the Fatigue Reactivity Mechanism.

The Fatigue Reactivity Mechanism describes the process by which recovery debt and lowered capacity increase reward sensitivity, reduce tolerance for delay or effort, and make fast, familiar, low-friction rewards feel more immediately valuable. The craving gains force because fatigue changes how much cognitive, emotional, and regulatory margin the system has available when the signal appears.

Under rested conditions, the nervous system often maintains greater flexibility around reward-related signals. A craving may still appear, but the system has more available bandwidth for reflection, contextual interpretation, competing priorities, uncertainty tolerance, and delayed response. Under fatigue, that margin narrows. The signal begins occupying more of the available system space because overall capacity has decreased.

The craving feels larger partly because the system feels smaller.

Fatigue should therefore be understood as lowered available function rather than laziness, weakness, or lack of effort. Recovery debt changes how much tolerance, patience, flexibility, and psychological distance the system can maintain when reward signals become active.

This is important because fatigue does not merely reduce energy in the narrow sense. It alters the economics of effort.

Ordinary demands become more expensive under recovery debt. Reflection costs more. Delay costs more. Uncertainty costs more. Cognitive switching costs more. Emotional regulation costs more. Complex decision-making costs more. The nervous system begins prioritizing efficiency because available capacity has narrowed.

Low-friction reward becomes more valuable when effort feels expensive.

Recovery debt refers to accumulated strain that has not yet been fully restored. The strain may involve cognitive load, emotional pressure, physical exertion, sleep disruption, sustained stress activation, prolonged vigilance, metabolic instability, excessive demand, insufficient restoration, or layered forms of unresolved fatigue. The important point here is not the precise source of exhaustion. The important point is that unresolved strain changes reward sensitivity.

A system operating under recovery debt evaluates effort differently.

The nervous system begins assigning greater importance to what appears easy, immediate, familiar, rapidly relieving, or cognitively inexpensive. Rewards associated with convenience, comfort, decompression, predictability, familiarity, sensory ease, or fast state change therefore gain additional salience because the system is attempting to reduce immediate burden under constrained capacity conditions.

The lower the capacity, the higher the value of ease.

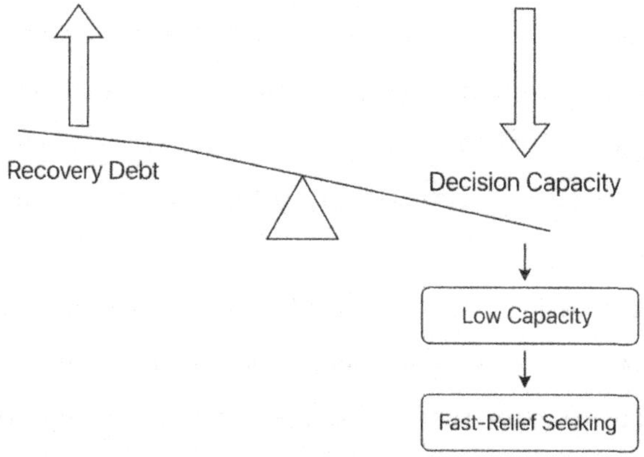

[Figure 13: Fatigue Reactivity Model]

The balancing model matters because it illustrates that recovery debt and decision capacity move in opposite directions. As unresolved strain increases, available functional margin decreases. The reduction in capacity increases sensitivity toward pathways associated with low-friction relief because the system has less tolerance for additional effort cost.

This helps explain why cravings often feel different under exhaustion than they do under rested conditions. The craving may not necessarily become more morally meaningful or biologically precise. It becomes more behaviorally persuasive because the surrounding system has less available bandwidth to absorb friction, delay, ambiguity, or internal conflict.

Fatigue reduces the room around the craving.

Reduced tolerance is central here because fatigue narrows the amount of discomfort, uncertainty, frustration, cognitive load, or emotional strain the system can comfortably carry. A person operating under recovery debt may therefore experience reward-related signals as more urgent because the nervous system has less surplus capacity available for sustained regulation.

The issue is not disappearance of agency. The issue is rising effort cost.

Fatigue does not erase choice. It raises the cost of distance.

This distinction prevents the chapter from drifting into deterministic language. A fatigued person does not become mechanically controlled by reward pathways. But the energetic and psychological cost of holding a craving at reflective distance often increases under exhaustion. The nervous system becomes increasingly motivated to reduce immediate strain efficiently.

Decision bandwidth narrows under fatigue for similar reasons. When capacity decreases, the system becomes less tolerant of prolonged deliberation, competing priorities, complex planning, or uncertain outcomes. Fast, familiar responses begin appearing more attractive because they reduce cognitive burden.

The system favors pathways requiring less negotiation.

This is one reason familiar reward loops often become especially persuasive during periods of fatigue. The pathway already exists. The anticipated outcome is known. The sequence requires less uncertainty and less cognitive assembly than novel or effort-intensive alternatives. The nervous system assigns value to familiarity because familiarity reduces processing demand.

Memory becomes more persuasive when capacity is low.

A known reward pathway feels psychologically efficient under fatigue because the system already understands the expected sequence. Familiarity lowers uncertainty. Predictability lowers cognitive cost. The nervous system gravitates toward what appears behaviorally easier because available margin is already constrained.

The craving therefore gains force partly through reduction of friction.

Fast-relief seeking emerges naturally under these conditions because the system increasingly values immediate reduction in discomfort, overload, heaviness, irritation, or effort burden. The anticipated reward does not need to involve dramatic pleasure. It may simply appear capable of making the current state easier to tolerate.

A fatigued system often seeks reduction before enjoyment.

This distinction is important because fatigue-related cravings are frequently misinterpreted as excessive indulgence or emotional weakness. But many fatigue-amplified reward signals organize around interruption of burden rather than pursuit of intense pleasure alone.

Comfort becomes valuable because strain feels expensive.

Convenience becomes valuable because planning feels expensive.

Familiarity becomes valuable because uncertainty feels expensive.

The craving gains emotional immediacy because the expected outcome appears capable of lowering present system cost quickly.

This helps explain why low-friction rewards become especially attractive under fatigue. A low-friction reward requires less preparation, less uncertainty, less waiting, less planning, less effort, and less cognitive negotiation. The nervous system increasingly prioritizes pathways associated with immediate accessibility because available functional capacity has narrowed.

Ease itself becomes rewarding under exhaustion.

This does not mean the system is irrational. Reduced capacity naturally changes motivational valuation. Under constrained conditions, the nervous system begins favoring what appears efficient relative to current available resources.

The lower the margin, the stronger the pull toward simplicity.

Fatigue also changes temporal preference. Under rested conditions, the system often tolerates delay more comfortably because sufficient margin exists to maintain distance between signal and response. Under exhaustion, delayed reward may feel psychologically less valuable because immediate relief carries greater importance.

The craving becomes more immediate because waiting feels heavier.

This immediacy can make reward signals feel unusually emotionally convincing. A familiar pathway associated with comfort, decompression, stimulation, or interruption of overload begins appearing behaviorally urgent because the system predicts rapid reduction in current burden.

Again, this does not require dramatic sensory reward. The anticipated value may involve softening of heaviness, interruption of cognitive fatigue, reduction in emotional irritability, lowering of effort demand, or temporary escape from accumulated strain.

Relief from exhaustion carries motivational weight.

Fatigue interacts strongly with cue association because familiar cues require less interpretive work than unfamiliar conditions. A repeated environment, routine, sensory exposure, transition point, or emotional context already associated with reward becomes increasingly persuasive under exhaustion because the pathway is easy to retrieve and easy to anticipate.

The nervous system prefers practiced routes when capacity narrows.

Memory intensifies this further because stored reward associations provide efficient predictive shortcuts. A familiar comfort-linked experience may feel especially compelling during fatigue because the system already trusts the pathway. The anticipated outcome appears reliable, recognizable, and behaviorally efficient relative to current available resources.

Fatigue increases the value of known relief.

This is one reason repeated reward loops can feel especially automatic during periods of exhaustion. The nervous system has reduced appetite for uncertainty under constrained capacity. Familiar pathways become increasingly attractive because they appear cognitively inexpensive and predictably relieving.

The craving narrows around what feels easiest to reach.

Fatigue also interacts with relief encoding directly. A tired system often seeks not merely pleasure, but reduction of effort burden, heaviness, irritability, overload, or internal strain. The craving may therefore carry expectation of immediate tolerability rather than intense sensory enjoyment.

The predicted reward says: make this state easier.

This distinction helps explain why fatigue-related cravings often feel emotionally compressed and urgent. The nervous system is not only pursuing reward in the abstract. It is attempting to reduce present state cost quickly under conditions of reduced available margin.

Fatigue therefore amplifies sensitivity to fast state change.

The relationship between strain and recovery capacity matters here because fatigue reflects mismatch between demand and restoration. When unresolved strain accumulates, the system loses flexibility. Reduced flexibility increases the emotional weight of immediate relief pathways because the nervous system has less available capacity for sustained effort or prolonged tension.

The craving becomes stronger because the system becomes narrower.

Importantly, this process does not make fatigue-related craving morally meaningful. A craving intensified by exhaustion is not evidence of weak character or failed discipline. The nervous system naturally recalibrates motivational priorities when available capacity declines.

A tired system does not value reward the same way a rested system does.

This also explains why cravings can fluctuate dramatically depending on recovery state even when environmental conditions remain similar. The same cue may feel relatively manageable under sufficient restoration and highly persuasive under recovery debt because the surrounding system conditions changed.

Fatigue alters salience by altering available margin.

The craving may therefore feel surprisingly immediate during periods of exhaustion because reduced tolerance, lowered decision bandwidth, increased effort cost, and heightened value of low-friction relief are operating simultaneously. The nervous system begins assigning greater importance to pathways associated with quick reduction in strain.

The signal gains force because capacity decreases.

This interaction becomes even stronger when fatigue combines with appetite pressure, glucose instability, stress load, emotional strain, or familiar reinforcement pathways. Multiple amplification systems converge. Broad depletion increases reward relevance. Fatigue increases effort sensitivity. Memory supplies familiar relief patterns. Cue association activates rapid anticipation. Relief encoding strengthens expected tolerability.

The resulting craving can feel unusually persuasive because several forms of pressure are operating at once.

Again, none of this requires self-control framing. The chapter is not arguing that fatigue removes agency or guarantees specific behavior. It is clarifying that recovery debt changes motivational conditions by narrowing capacity and increasing the value of fast, familiar, low-friction reward pathways.

The cost structure of the system changes under exhaustion.

Seen clearly, fatigue reactivity makes craving more understandable and less morally confusing. The craving becomes amplified because reduced capacity increases reward sensitivity while lowering tolerance for friction, delay, uncertainty, or sustained effort. Fast relief gains emotional importance because available margin has narrowed.

A craving intensified by recovery debt is therefore not proof of weak discipline. It is a reward signal amplified by reduced tolerance, higher effort cost, lowered capacity, and increased sensitivity to immediate relief under constrained conditions.

The nervous system prioritizes ease when carrying too much unresolved strain.

Stress Salience Mechanism

Stress changes craving intensity by changing what becomes salient. A reward signal that might remain relatively mild under lower-pressure conditions can become more noticeable, more emotionally persuasive, and more difficult to hold at distance when stress load rises. The object itself may not fundamentally change. What changes is the nervous system's relationship to relief, decompression, interruption, familiarity, and immediate state change.

Stress increases the value of relief.

This distinction matters because stress-related cravings are often interpreted through moral language rather than systems language. A person under high strain may experience stronger reward pull and conclude that discipline weakened, restraint collapsed, or self-control disappeared. But stress changes the operating conditions under which reward signals are evaluated. The nervous system reorganizes motivational priority when internal pressure rises.

A stressed system does not weigh relief neutrally.

This is the Stress Salience Mechanism.

The Stress Salience Mechanism describes the process by which stress load increases the perceived importance of immediate reward by narrowing tolerance, reducing available margin, increasing relief value, and making rapid regulation feel more behaviorally relevant. The craving gains force because the nervous system becomes increasingly attentive to anything associated with interruption of pressure, decompression, familiarity, or emotional softening.

Stress therefore functions as a salience amplifier.

Under lower stress conditions, a reward cue may remain psychologically moderate because the surrounding system state still contains sufficient flexibility, margin, and tolerance. The nervous system can evaluate the signal without assigning urgent importance to it. Under higher stress load, the same cue may feel emotionally larger because the anticipated relief associated with the reward becomes increasingly valuable.

The reward gains weight because the pressure around it increases.

Stress load can emerge from many overlapping conditions: sustained cognitive demand, emotional strain, uncertainty, vigilance, overload, social tension, unresolved pressure, environmental instability, prolonged responsibility, accumulated frustration, time compression, decision burden, interrupted recovery, or persistent activation without sufficient downshift. The specific source matters less here than the effect stress has on motivational organization.

Stress narrows the system around relief relevance.

The nervous system under strain becomes increasingly attentive to signals associated with reduction of pressure. A familiar reward pathway linked with decompression, interruption, comfort, distraction, stimulation, sensory certainty, or emotional softening therefore becomes more salient because the system assigns higher value to possible regulation.

The craving feels more important because relief feels more important.

Importantly, this process does not require dramatic pleasure-seeking. Many stress-amplified cravings organize around interruption of strain rather than pursuit of intense enjoyment. The anticipated value may involve temporary quieting, reduction of internal friction, emotional softening, cognitive interruption, familiar sensory predictability, or brief decompression from overload.

Relief becomes motivationally heavy under pressure.

Stress does not create every craving, but it changes the emotional size of reward signals already present. A familiar sensory cue, remembered comfort pathway, or anticipated decompression sequence becomes behaviorally amplified because the nervous system increasingly prioritizes anything associated with reduced burden.

The higher the strain, the louder the relief pathway may become.

Narrowed tolerance is central to this process because stress reduces available margin for additional discomfort, ambiguity, delay, emotional friction, uncertainty, frustration, or effort. The system becomes less able to comfortably absorb unresolved pressure. Immediate reward therefore becomes more behaviorally attractive because it appears capable of changing the current state quickly.

Stress reduces the room around discomfort.

Under elevated strain, waiting feels heavier. Friction feels sharper. Emotional ambiguity feels more expensive. Additional demands feel more intrusive. The nervous system begins assigning greater value to pathways associated with fast interruption of pressure because available tolerance has narrowed.

The craving gains urgency because the system loses margin.

This does not imply disappearance of agency or collapse of conscious decision-making. The issue is not absence of capacity, but reduction in available flexibility. The cost of carrying unresolved tension increases under stress load. Immediate reward becomes more behaviorally persuasive because relief appears emotionally efficient relative to the current condition.

Stress increases the appeal of fast state change.

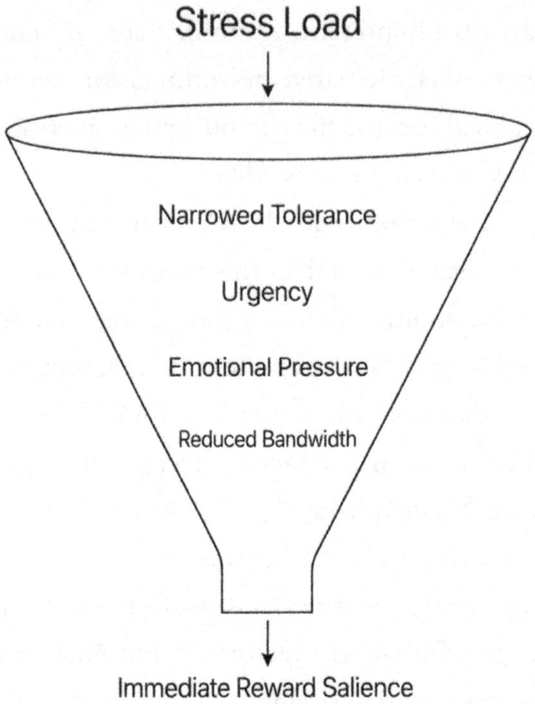

[Figure 14: Stress Salience Funnel]

The funnel model matters because it illustrates how stress compresses behavioral flexibility toward immediate regulation pathways. As internal load increases, tolerance narrows, emotional pressure rises, bandwidth decreases, and reward salience intensifies. The nervous system begins orienting more strongly toward what appears rapidly relieving because the surrounding system state becomes increasingly difficult to sustain.

Stress funnels attention toward relief.

Immediate relief preference develops naturally under these conditions because the nervous system increasingly values speed when carrying elevated pressure. A delayed or uncertain reward may feel less behaviorally useful than one associated with rapid decompression, interruption, or emotional softening.

Immediacy becomes valuable when tolerance narrows.

This helps explain why familiar rewards often feel unusually compelling during stress even when the actual object itself has not changed. The nervous system is not evaluating reward in isolation. It is evaluating reward while carrying heightened internal load. The anticipated outcome becomes emotionally amplified because the present condition feels increasingly burdensome.

The craving says: reduce this state quickly.

Stress also alters attentional organization. Under lower-pressure conditions, competing priorities, reflective distance, and broader context may remain easier to maintain. Under elevated stress, attention narrows around pathways associated with immediate regulation because the system increasingly prioritizes reduction of current strain.

Relief becomes more visible under stress.

This increased visibility is what makes reward salience feel psychologically convincing during periods of overload. The reward cue stands out more because the nervous system is actively searching for interruption of pressure. The craving gains emotional force because the anticipated state change feels behaviorally relevant.

A stressed system notices relief faster.

Reward can therefore function as a temporary regulation substitute under stress load. A craving may intensify because the anticipated response appears capable of briefly reducing emotional tension, cognitive overload, irritability, internal compression, restlessness, heaviness, or sustained vigilance. The response becomes meaningful because it appears to shift the state.

The issue is not whether the regulation is perfect, complete, or lasting. The issue is that the nervous system predicts meaningful interruption of strain.

Temporary decompression can become highly persuasive under sustained pressure.

This distinction prevents the chapter from drifting into moralized "stress eating" language. The systems question is not whether stress-related reward seeking is virtuous or problematic. The systems question is how stress changes motivational weighting around relief-associated pathways.

Stress does not make reward stronger by magic. It makes relief more valuable.

This also explains why familiar comfort-associated patterns often become especially persuasive during periods of high strain. Memory supplies previously learned regulation pathways. Cue association activates them quickly. Reinforcement history increases confidence in the anticipated effect. Stress amplifies their motivational relevance because decompression feels increasingly important.

Memory provides the route. Stress increases the urgency of taking it.

A familiar sensory experience linked with emotional interruption or temporary quieting may therefore become highly salient under stress because the nervous system already recognizes the sequence as potentially regulating. The anticipated outcome gains force because relief value has increased.

The craving becomes emotionally persuasive because pressure changes prediction.

Stress interacts strongly with cue association because familiar environments, routines, transition points, emotional states, or sensory exposures already connected with prior decompression become easier to activate under strain. A repeated evening routine, a familiar screen environment, a certain social context, or a specific sensory cue may trigger stronger craving under stress because the nervous system associates the context with interruption of pressure.

The cue becomes louder when strain increases.

Stress also interacts powerfully with fatigue reactivity. Fatigue lowers available capacity while stress increases internal load. Together, they narrow tolerance dramatically. Reflection becomes more expensive.

Delay becomes harder to sustain. Low-friction reward pathways become increasingly attractive because both exhaustion and pressure increase the value of immediate relief.

The combination compresses the system toward ease and interruption.

Glucose urgency can intensify this further because unstable energy availability combined with stress load increases both physiological and emotional pressure simultaneously. The nervous system may then assign extremely high salience to pathways associated with rapid restoration, stabilization, or sensory certainty because multiple amplification systems are operating together.

The craving gains force from convergence.

Under these layered conditions, a reward signal may feel unusually immediate not because the object itself is inherently overwhelming, but because stress, fatigue, instability, and learned relief pathways are collectively increasing the perceived importance of rapid regulation.

Again, this does not make the craving morally meaningful. A stressed system does not evaluate reward the same way a lower-pressure system does. The nervous system naturally prioritizes pathways associated with reduction of strain when tolerance narrows and internal load rises.

Pressure changes motivational hierarchy.

Importantly, the anticipated relief does not need to be dramatic to become reinforcing. Even temporary interruption, mild decompression, familiar sensory predictability, cognitive quieting, emotional softening, or reduction of tension can acquire substantial motivational value under high stress because the surrounding system state already feels expensive to maintain.

The reward becomes valuable because the strain feels costly.

This also helps explain why stress-amplified cravings often feel emotionally disproportionate relative to the actual object involved. The emotional intensity belongs partly to the stress state itself. The craving carries amplified weight because the nervous system is attempting to reduce accumulated pressure quickly.

The signal becomes more urgent because the system becomes less tolerant.

Importantly, stress-driven craving should not be confused with weakness, lack of discipline, or defective self-regulation. The nervous system is functioning adaptively within a high-load environment. Increased salience surrounding relief pathways reflects altered motivational organization under strain, not moral failure.

A stressed system prioritizes interruption differently than a rested one.

Seen clearly, stress salience makes craving more understandable and less morally confusing. The craving becomes amplified because stress narrows tolerance, reduces available margin, increases relief value, and heightens attentional sensitivity toward rapid regulation pathways.

The nervous system becomes more responsive to immediate reward because the current state feels increasingly difficult to sustain.

A craving intensified by stress load is therefore not proof of weak discipline. It is a reward signal amplified by reduced margin, elevated internal pressure, narrowed tolerance, and increased motivational value assigned to decompression, interruption, familiarity, and fast relief under strain.

The system moves toward relief because pressure changes what feels behaviorally important.

Sleep Debt Sensitivity Mechanism

Sleep debt changes craving sensitivity because poor recovery strains multiple regulation layers at once. A craving that might remain interpretable, moderate, or psychologically manageable under sufficient recovery can feel more frequent, more urgent, more emotionally charged, and more difficult to hold at distance when sleep loss accumulates. The reward signal itself may not fundamentally change in structure, but the system receiving the signal changes substantially under insufficient recovery.

The nervous system under sleep debt operates with reduced margin.

This distinction matters because cravings during periods of poor recovery are often interpreted as personal inconsistency or failed discipline rather than as altered system conditions. A person may experience stronger reward pull, shorter delay tolerance, heightened emotional urgency, or increased food salience after insufficient sleep and assume something morally meaningful has changed. But sleep debt modifies how multiple regulation systems interact simultaneously.

Recovery strain changes motivational weighting.

This is the Sleep Debt Sensitivity Mechanism.

The Sleep Debt Sensitivity Mechanism describes the process by which insufficient recovery increases craving sensitivity by raising appetite pressure, reducing emotional regulation capacity, increasing impulse pressure, heightening reward salience, and lowering the system's margin for clear interpretation. Cravings gain force because multiple stabilizing layers become strained simultaneously under inadequate recovery conditions.

Sleep therefore functions as part of regulation capacity rather than merely absence of wakefulness.

When sleep is shortened, fragmented, poorly timed, inconsistent, or insufficiently restorative, the system carries unresolved strain into the next cycle. The nervous system begins operating under accumulated recovery loss. Appetite regulation, emotional tolerance, cognitive flexibility, stress responsiveness, reward valuation, and decision bandwidth all become more vulnerable to amplification effects because available margin narrows across several systems simultaneously.

Poor recovery increases background pressure before the craving even appears.

A reward cue encountered under sufficient recovery may therefore feel entirely different when encountered under sleep debt. The same sensory exposure, familiar pathway, emotional state, or contextual trigger may become substantially more persuasive because the surrounding nervous system is carrying more strain and less flexibility.

The craving becomes larger because recovery margin becomes smaller.

Importantly, sleep debt does not create every craving. The system already contains learned reward pathways, memory associations, cue structures, reinforcement patterns, anticipated relief sequences, and metabolic pressures. Poor recovery amplifies those systems by lowering tolerance and increasing salience across multiple layers at once.

Sleep debt lowers the threshold for many signals simultaneously.

The nervous system under inadequate recovery becomes more sensitive to what appears immediately regulating, emotionally softening, rapidly restoring, cognitively interrupting, or behaviorally easy. Familiar reward pathways gain additional leverage because the system is operating with reduced reserve capacity.

Recovery loss increases the value of immediacy.

This interaction helps explain why cravings often feel more frequent under sleep debt even when external conditions remain relatively similar. More internal states begin functioning as pressure states. More environmental cues become behaviorally noticeable. More reward pathways feel emotionally relevant because the system has less recovery margin available to absorb friction, delay, instability, uncertainty, or strain.

A tired system detects relief opportunities more aggressively.

Sleep debt also amplifies appetite pressure because poor recovery changes overall food relevance. The nervous system under insufficient restoration often operates with greater compensation pressure surrounding intake, energy restoration, and rapid reward accessibility. The result is not necessarily constant hunger in a simplistic sense, but increased motivational responsiveness toward reward-related signals.

Food relevance rises when recovery falls.

This helps explain why reward cues often feel more emotionally persuasive after inadequate sleep. Appetite pressure and reward salience begin overlapping more heavily because the system is already operating under strain. Familiar sensory pathways associated with comfort, stimulation, convenience, speed, or decompression therefore acquire additional motivational weight.

The craving gains force because restoration feels increasingly important.

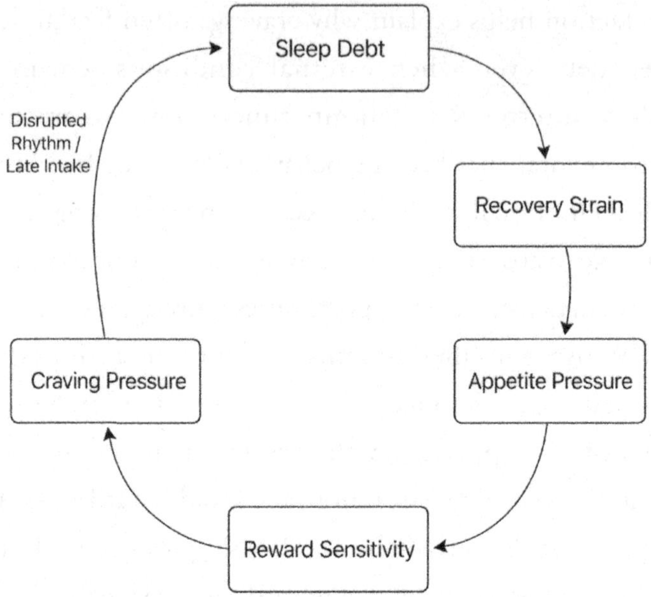

[Figure 15: Sleep Debt Sensitivity Loop]

The loop model matters because it illustrates how poor recovery amplifies several interacting systems simultaneously. Sleep debt increases recovery strain. Recovery strain raises appetite pressure, emotional sensitivity, fatigue reactivity, stress responsiveness, and reward salience. Increased craving pressure can then contribute to further rhythm disruption, late intake, irregular regulation, or continued strain accumulation.

The system becomes easier to activate when recovery weakens.

Emotional regulation strain becomes especially important under insufficient recovery because emotional states often feel sharper, heavier, or more difficult to absorb when nervous system restoration is incomplete. Frustration tolerance narrows. Irritability rises more quickly. Emotional friction becomes more behaviorally expensive. Internal pressure states acquire greater emotional weight because the system has reduced stabilizing capacity available.

The emotional cost of carrying strain increases under sleep debt.

Cravings may therefore intensify because the anticipated reward appears capable of softening emotional pressure temporarily. The nervous system begins assigning higher value to pathways associated with decompression, comfort, interruption, distraction, familiarity, or rapid emotional easing because emotional regulation itself becomes more difficult to sustain under inadequate recovery.

Poor recovery increases the appeal of emotional interruption.

This process should not be confused with lack of character or failed discipline. Emotional strain under sleep debt reflects altered regulation conditions, not moral weakness. The nervous system simply operates differently when recovery capacity narrows across multiple layers simultaneously.

Impulse pressure changes for similar reasons. Impulse pressure does not mean loss of agency or inability to choose. It means the distance between signal and response becomes shorter because reflective bandwidth, emotional margin, tolerance for discomfort, and decision flexibility are reduced under recovery strain.

The signal reaches action more quickly when margin narrows.

A craving that might remain psychologically manageable under adequate recovery can feel substantially more immediate after poor sleep because the nervous system has less available room for delay, contextual interpretation, uncertainty tolerance, or sustained reflective distance.

Sleep debt compresses the space around the craving.

This compression changes the emotional texture of reward signals. Immediate relief pathways begin appearing more behaviorally valuable because prolonged strain feels harder to carry under reduced recovery conditions.

Waiting feels heavier under sleep debt.

Friction feels sharper.

Immediacy gains emotional value because tolerance decreases.

Reward sensitivity also increases because the nervous system under insufficient recovery assigns greater motivational importance to familiar pathways associated with fast restoration, comfort, stimulation, or low-friction state change. Sensory intensity, convenience, predictability, speed, and familiarity become increasingly persuasive because the system values efficiency under constrained conditions.

A poorly recovered system prioritizes what feels rapidly regulating.

This does not necessarily mean the reward itself becomes objectively stronger. The salience changes because the system state changes. Familiar rewards gain emotional leverage because the nervous system is operating with less flexibility, lower reserve capacity, and increased sensitivity to relief-related possibilities.

The lower the recovery margin, the higher the value of fast relief.

Fatigue reactivity intensifies this further because sleep debt contributes directly to reduced available capacity. Reflection becomes more expensive. Effort tolerance narrows. Planning feels heavier. Familiar pathways require less uncertainty and less cognitive assembly, so they become increasingly attractive under recovery strain.

Poor recovery increases the motivational value of ease.

A familiar reward pathway therefore feels especially persuasive during sleep debt because memory supplies a known route toward anticipated relief while reduced capacity increases the value of low-friction regulation. The nervous system increasingly favors what appears behaviorally efficient relative to current available resources.

The craving feels convincing because the pathway feels easy to reach.

Stress salience interacts powerfully with this process as well. Sleep debt often increases stress sensitivity while simultaneously lowering emotional margin. The result is heightened attentional responsiveness toward pathways associated with interruption of pressure. Stress feels more intrusive under inadequate recovery because tolerance narrows and regulatory flexibility decreases.

A stressed, sleep-deprived system assigns high value to decompression.

This combination can make cravings feel unusually emotionally immediate because several amplification systems converge simultaneously. Appetite pressure rises. Fatigue reduces capacity. Emotional regulation narrows. Stress sensitivity increases. Reward salience intensifies. Familiar memory pathways become more persuasive. Cue association activates more easily.

The signal begins carrying multiple layers of urgency at once.

Glucose urgency may also become more behaviorally relevant under poor recovery because unstable energy availability often feels more difficult to tolerate when the nervous system is already strained. Fog, heaviness, irritability, shakiness, reduced patience, or fluctuating energy states become more emotionally significant because overall recovery capacity has declined.

Poor recovery magnifies instability.

The craving may therefore feel like one unified urgent demand even when multiple overlapping systems are amplifying it simultaneously. Appetite pressure, fatigue reactivity, stress salience, emotional strain, memory activation, cue association, glucose urgency, and anticipated relief may all be contributing to the signal at once.

This is one reason cravings under sleep debt are often harder to interpret clearly.

The nervous system loses interpretive clarity when too many amplification layers become active simultaneously. The craving feels singular and emotionally authoritative even though several interacting systems are contributing pressure underneath it.

The system becomes louder and less differentiated under recovery strain.

Importantly, this does not mean sleep debt produces irrationality or total loss of regulation. The point is more structural: insufficient recovery lowers overall margin, increases reward sensitivity, shortens delay tolerance, heightens emotional responsiveness, and amplifies multiple forms of motivational pressure simultaneously.

The cost structure of regulation changes under poor recovery.

This helps explain why cravings often appear more frequently during periods of insufficient sleep. More cues become salient. More internal states function as pressure states. More reward pathways appear behaviorally relevant because the system is operating with reduced resilience and higher background strain.

The nervous system scans more aggressively for relief when recovery is incomplete.

Again, none of this requires moral framing. A craving intensified by sleep debt is not evidence of weak discipline, lack of character, or defective self-control. The system under inadequate recovery conditions simply evaluates reward, relief, effort, and emotional pressure differently than a sufficiently recovered system does.

Recovery capacity changes motivational organization.

Seen clearly, sleep debt sensitivity makes craving more understandable and less morally confusing. Poor recovery amplifies appetite pressure, emotional strain, fatigue reactivity, stress sensitivity, reward salience, and impulse pressure simultaneously. The craving gains force because multiple stabilizing systems are carrying unresolved strain at once.

The nervous system moves more quickly toward relief when recovery margin narrows.

A craving intensified by insufficient sleep is therefore not proof of weak discipline. It is a reward signal amplified by reduced recovery capacity, increased emotional pressure, narrowed tolerance, heightened reward sensitivity, shortened reflective distance, and the system's attempt to restore stability under strained conditions.

Availability Friction Mechanism

Craving changes not only through internal pressure, memory, reinforcement, fatigue, stress, or appetite instability, but also through exposure frequency and response effort. A reward pathway that is repeatedly visible, easily accessible, familiar, fast, and low in friction has more opportunities to activate than one that rarely enters attention or requires substantial effort to pursue. Availability therefore shapes craving frequency not because it forces behavior, but because it changes how often the loop has a chance to run.

This distinction matters because cravings are often interpreted as though they emerge entirely from internal desire or personal weakness while the surrounding environment remains psychologically neutral. But repeated exposure changes activation probability. Accessibility changes response effort. Familiarity changes readiness. The nervous system does not encounter all rewards under identical structural conditions.

Some pathways are encountered constantly.

Some pathways are easy to complete.

Some pathways repeatedly reactivate because the environment keeps presenting them.

This is the Availability Friction Mechanism.

The Availability Friction Mechanism describes the process by which repeated exposure, low response effort, and easy access increase cue contact and reinforcement opportunities, making craving loops more frequent and easier to activate. Availability changes the frequency of activation opportunities, while friction changes the effort required for the sequence to continue from cue to response.

Availability does not create a command. It creates another chance for the loop to run.

This difference is important because exposure alone does not eliminate agency. The environment does not mechanically control behavior. But environmental structure influences how often cues appear, how rapidly reward prediction activates, how much effort a response requires, and how frequently reinforcement opportunities occur across time.

Frequency shapes familiarity.

Familiarity shapes readiness.

Repeated opportunities shape loop strength.

Availability begins with exposure. A cue cannot activate unless contact occurs. The more often a reward-associated object, environment, routine, sensory signal, or behavioral pathway enters awareness, the more frequently the nervous system has opportunities to reactivate learned prediction. Even low-intensity exposures matter when repeated consistently across time.

The nervous system learns through repetition density as much as through intensity.

A reward does not need to produce dramatic emotional force every time to strengthen familiarity. Repeated low-level contact can gradually normalize the pathway, increase salience, and strengthen response readiness simply because the sequence is encountered frequently.

Frequency accumulates structurally.

A visible reward pathway has more activation opportunities than an invisible one.

This is especially important because craving often feels spontaneous even when activation probability has been repeatedly increased through environmental contact. A person may experience recurring urges in a highly exposed environment and interpret the experience as purely internal when the nervous system has actually been receiving continuous low-level cue activation across time.

Exposure increases the number of times prediction can begin.

Availability therefore changes the architecture of opportunity. A reward-associated cue that appears repeatedly throughout ordinary routines acquires repeated chances to reactivate memory, anticipated relief, reward salience, sensory prediction, or reinforcement expectation.

Repeated exposure increases pattern accessibility.

Low-friction reward access intensifies this further because the distance between cue and response becomes short, familiar, rapid, and easy to complete. Friction refers to the amount of effort, delay, planning, uncertainty, preparation, tolerance, or resistance required for a pathway to continue toward completion.

Low friction shortens the pathway between wanting and obtaining.

A low-friction reward is behaviorally easy to reach. It requires minimal interruption of momentum. The pathway already exists. The sequence is familiar. The response can occur quickly and predictably with little uncertainty or planning burden.

Ease changes repetition frequency before it changes identity.

This distinction matters because highly accessible rewards often become more behaviorally central simply because they are easier to repeat consistently. Repetition density increases because the response cost remains low.

The easiest pathway is not always the strongest pathway; it is often the most repeated one.

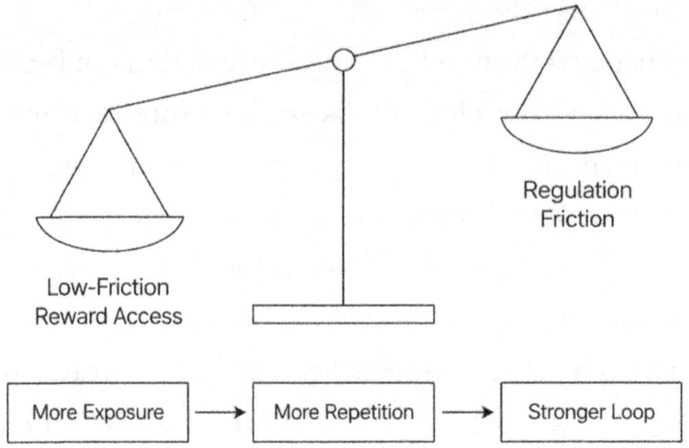

[Figure 16: Availability and Friction Balance]

Repeated cue contact becomes especially powerful over time because familiarity reduces activation requirements. The nervous system does not need dramatic emotional intensity to strengthen a pathway. Frequent low-level exposures can gradually increase readiness because each contact slightly reinforces recognition, anticipation, memory linkage, or response expectation.

Small repetitions accumulate into structural familiarity.

A cue encountered occasionally may remain relatively neutral. A cue encountered repeatedly within ordinary environments gains increasing predictive relevance simply because the nervous system begins recognizing it as part of recurring behavioral structure.

The pathway becomes easier to retrieve because it is repeatedly rehearsed.

This process helps explain why craving frequency often reflects environmental repetition as much as internal intensity. A reward repeatedly encountered throughout ordinary routines naturally receives more opportunities for activation than one rarely entering awareness.

Availability changes loop frequency through repetition opportunity.

Friction becomes equally important because reward pathways and regulation pathways rarely exist under identical effort conditions. If reward is immediate, familiar, accessible, and low effort while regulation requires delay, planning, uncertainty tolerance, emotional bandwidth, recovery capacity, or sustained discomfort tolerance, the nervous system may repeatedly gravitate toward the lower-friction route.

Friction imbalance shapes behavioral probability.

This does not require moral interpretation. The nervous system generally favors pathways requiring less effort when strain, fatigue, stress, sleep debt, emotional overload, or reduced capacity increase the perceived cost of friction-heavy alternatives.

The system under pressure becomes increasingly sensitive to effort cost.

A low-friction reward pathway therefore becomes especially persuasive under constrained conditions because it appears capable of delivering state change quickly with minimal expenditure of already-limited resources.

Ease gains value when capacity narrows.

Importantly, regulation friction does not only mean self-control effort. Regulation may require waiting, uncertainty tolerance, emotional endurance, preparation, flexibility, reflective distance, energy availability, cognitive bandwidth, or tolerance for unresolved discomfort. Under low-capacity conditions, those demands become increasingly expensive.

The nervous system under strain values immediacy differently than a rested system does.

Environment therefore shapes loop frequency not by removing agency, but by continuously altering cue density, response effort, activation probability, and reinforcement opportunity across time.

Structure influences repetition before repetition influences identity.

This distinction helps prevent moral overinterpretation of frequently activated cravings. A loop repeatedly activated within low-friction conditions may strengthen rapidly simply because the environment repeatedly supplies opportunities for the sequence to run.

Repeated opportunity accelerates familiarity.

Repeated familiarity accelerates automaticity.

Automaticity lowers future activation threshold.

Availability also interacts strongly with cue association because visible and repeated exposures increase the number of times contextual prediction can become linked to reward expectation. A familiar environment repeatedly paired with anticipated relief, stimulation, comfort, decompression, or sensory reward gradually strengthens contextual activation.

The environment begins carrying predictive weight.

This does not mean every visible cue becomes behaviorally dominant. But increased cue contact statistically increases opportunities for memory reactivation, reward anticipation, reinforcement repetition, and response completion.

More exposure creates more chances for activation.

Availability further interacts with memory reactivation because familiar reward pathways remain easier to retrieve when environmental cues repeatedly refresh associative networks. The nervous system does not need to reconstruct the pathway each time from the beginning. Familiarity keeps the sequence psychologically accessible.

Repeated contact preserves pathway readiness.

This helps explain why certain cravings feel chronically close to activation in highly exposed environments. The pathway rarely has time to become psychologically distant because repeated environmental contact continuously refreshes recognition and anticipated reward structures.

The signal remains near the surface because exposure remains continuous.

Fatigue reactivity intensifies the influence of low-friction reward because tired systems assign higher value to convenience, familiarity, low effort, and rapid state change. Under reduced capacity, rewards requiring minimal planning or tolerance become especially attractive because effort itself feels more expensive.

Low-friction rewards become more persuasive when energy is limited.

Stress salience amplifies the same process. A stressed nervous system values rapid decompression, interruption, predictability, and relief. When immediate rewards remain highly accessible during periods of elevated strain, the pathway gains additional motivational relevance because the environment supplies quick routes toward anticipated state change.

Stress increases the value of immediate accessibility.

Sleep debt sensitivity further narrows margin. Poor recovery lowers tolerance, increases reward salience, reduces reflective distance, and heightens impulse pressure. Under those conditions, friction-heavy regulation pathways feel increasingly expensive while low-friction rewards feel increasingly behaviorally efficient.

Reduced recovery increases sensitivity to ease.

Availability also interacts with appetite pressure and glucose urgency. Under conditions of perceived scarcity, unstable fuel availability, fatigue, irritability, or heightened appetite relevance, visible and accessible rewards acquire additional salience because the nervous system already values restoration, immediacy, or rapid state change more strongly.

Pressure amplifies the attractiveness of accessible reward.

This does not mean availability creates cravings in isolation. Environmental structure interacts continuously with internal state, reinforcement history, memory architecture, emotional strain, metabolic conditions, and reward prediction systems already developed throughout the book.

The environment shapes opportunity rather than destiny.

Importantly, this chapter is not proposing environmental-control ideology. The point is not that accessible rewards must be removed, feared, restricted, or morally condemned. Environmental structure is being interpreted descriptively, not prescriptively.

Availability is not a moral contaminant.

Low-friction reward access does not prove weakness, lack of discipline, or defective self-control. It changes exposure frequency, repetition density, response effort, and reinforcement opportunity. Over time, those structural conditions influence how often loops activate and how familiar pathways become.

The loop strengthens through repetition opportunity as much as through intensity.

This distinction reduces confusion because highly repeated cravings often feel personally revealing when they may partly reflect environmental repetition structure. A pathway repeatedly exposed, easily accessible, behaviorally efficient, and low in friction naturally acquires more opportunities for reinforcement than a pathway rarely encountered or difficult to complete.

Friction changes frequency before it changes identity.

Seen clearly, availability and friction make craving patterns more understandable without moralizing them. A frequently activated craving loop is not necessarily evidence of weak discipline or failed character. It may reflect repeated cue contact, low response effort, preserved familiarity, high environmental exposure, reduced regulation margin, and continuous opportunities for reinforcement.

The nervous system repeats what remains repeatedly available.

The pathway becomes stronger partly because the environment keeps offering chances for activation, prediction, response, and reinforcement to occur again. Availability changes how often the signal appears. Friction changes how easily the sequence continues. Together, they shape how frequently craving loops reactivate across time and how familiar those loops eventually become within the larger architecture of reward prediction and reinforcement.

Pattern Recognition Mechanism

Cravings become harder to interpret when every craving is treated as the same kind of signal. A craving may feel urgent, emotionally charged, repetitive, highly specific, or difficult to ignore, but those qualities do not automatically indicate the same source each time. The nervous system can produce similar intensities through very different structures. Without differentiation, distinct craving patterns collapse into one undifferentiated experience, and interpretation becomes increasingly confused.

This confusion often produces moral explanation in place of structural explanation. A recurring craving may be interpreted as weakness. A situational craving may be interpreted as loss of control. A compensatory craving may be interpreted as emotional failure. A reinforced loop may be mistaken for simple hunger. When different signal structures are treated as interchangeable, the craving loses interpretive clarity.

The signal becomes emotionally loaded because its structure remains invisible.

This is the Pattern Recognition Mechanism.

The Pattern Recognition Mechanism describes the process of distinguishing different craving structures so a craving can be interpreted according to its source pattern rather than collapsed into a single moral, emotional, or hunger-based explanation. Recognition does not reduce craving to rigid categories or fixed identities. It improves clarity by separating distinct forms of amplification, prediction, reinforcement, context activation, and pressure compensation.

Not every craving is built the same way.

This distinction matters because craving is often discussed as though it represents one unified phenomenon. But the nervous system can generate cravings through different combinations of appetite pressure, cue association, memory activation, emotional strain, fatigue reactivity, stress salience, reward expectation, environmental exposure, reinforcement history, and perceived relief value. The resulting experiences may feel superficially similar while emerging from very different structures.

Recognition therefore changes interpretation rather than moral judgment.

A craving becomes easier to understand when its organizing pattern becomes visible.

Four broad craving patterns help clarify this distinction: occasional cravings, situational cravings, compensatory cravings, and reinforced craving loops. These are not diagnoses or fixed identities. They are interpretive structures that help distinguish how different craving signals become organized.

Occasional cravings are periodic signals that appear without strong repetitive reinforcement, narrow context dependence, or deeply established automaticity. They may reflect ordinary desire, sensory curiosity, novelty, remembered enjoyment, temporary appetite relevance, or transient reward expectation. These cravings often remain relatively flexible because they are not heavily embedded within repeated reinforcement structures.

An occasional craving does not necessarily indicate instability.

A person may experience desire for a particular sensory experience, familiar taste, seasonal association, or pleasurable reward without the craving becoming central, repetitive, or highly automatic. The nervous system naturally generates intermittent reward interest as part of ordinary predictive behavior.

Occasional does not mean meaningless. It means structurally lighter.

Situational cravings differ because they become strongly linked to context. Time of day, environment, routines, transitions, sensory exposures, social settings, screens, smells, routes, or repeated circumstances activate the signal through learned association. The craving becomes easier to understand once the contextual structure becomes visible.

The context carries prediction forward before conscious reflection fully forms.

A particular evening routine may repeatedly activate a familiar reward expectation. A certain work transition may become associated with decompression. A screen environment may increase sensory anticipation. A social setting may reactivate prior reward memory. The craving emerges not necessarily because the object itself suddenly became biologically urgent, but because the surrounding conditions reactivate learned prediction.

Situational cravings reveal the power of context-linked expectation.

Compensatory cravings organize differently because they emerge more strongly under conditions of pressure, instability, depletion, or reduced tolerance. Fatigue, stress load, sleep debt, glucose instability, emotional strain, boredom, restriction pressure, appetite pressure, overload, or unresolved discomfort increase the value of relief, stimulation, interruption, familiarity, or rapid regulation. The craving gains intensity because the nervous system is attempting to offset an uncomfortable state.

The signal is not only pursuing reward. It is responding to pressure.

Compensatory cravings therefore often carry strong expectation of state change. The anticipated outcome may involve emotional softening, decompression, sensory interruption, rapid stabilization, reduced heaviness, increased alertness, lowered tension, or temporary tolerability. The craving becomes emotionally persuasive because the current state feels increasingly expensive to sustain.

Pressure increases the value of relief pathways.

Reinforced craving loops emerge through repeated pairing between cue, anticipation, response, reward or relief, and reinforcement across time. The nervous system learns the sequence through repetition, lowering activation threshold and increasing automaticity. These cravings often feel highly familiar, rapidly activated, and contextually predictable because the pathway has already been practiced extensively.

Repetition increases retrieval efficiency.

A cue that once produced mild interest may eventually activate rapid craving because the sequence has become structurally reinforced through repeated association. The nervous system recognizes the pattern quickly and restores the expected pathway with increasing speed and reduced friction.

Familiar loops activate faster because the architecture already exists.

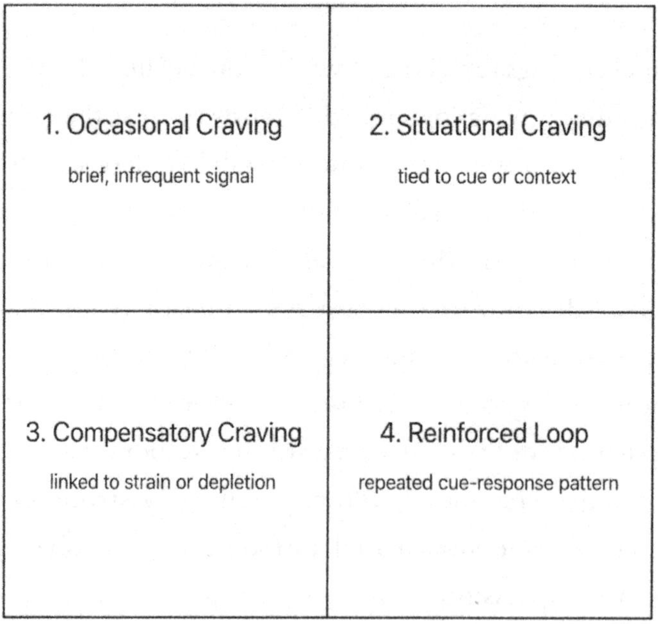

[Figure 17: Craving Pattern Categories]

The categories matter because they separate structure without turning craving into pathology. The purpose is not to create personality types, diagnostic labels, or rigid classifications. A single craving can contain multiple overlapping patterns simultaneously. A situational craving may become reinforced over time. A compensatory craving may attach to familiar contextual cues. An occasional craving may later become more repetitive under reinforcement or stress amplification.

Patterns overlap because systems interact.

This is important because human behavior rarely organizes itself into perfectly isolated categories. The nervous system operates through layered interaction. Appetite pressure may intensify a situational craving. Sleep debt may amplify a compensatory craving. Reinforcement history may strengthen context-linked activation. Emotional strain may increase the salience of familiar reward memory.

Recognition improves interpretation by separating the dominant structure rather than demanding perfect purity.

A craving does not need to fit one category completely to become more understandable.

Occasional cravings are especially important to distinguish because not every reward-oriented signal indicates instability, reinforcement pathology, or unresolved pressure. The nervous system naturally generates intermittent desire, curiosity, sensory interest, novelty seeking, and context-linked pleasure anticipation as part of ordinary adaptive behavior.

Not every craving carries heavy reinforcement architecture.

Without this distinction, ordinary reward interest can become unnecessarily moralized or overinterpreted. The existence of desire alone does not automatically imply compulsion, dysfunction, or emotional collapse. Occasional cravings may remain relatively flexible precisely because they are not strongly embedded within repeated cue-response-reward structures.

Situational cravings clarify how strongly context organizes anticipation. A person may feel confused by recurring urges appearing at similar times or in similar settings and interpret the experience as evidence of poor discipline. But often the structure becomes more understandable once contextual prediction becomes visible.

The environment may be activating the signal before deliberate intention fully forms.

Repeated evening routines, work transitions, social rituals, sensory exposures, entertainment environments, familiar stores, driving routes, seasonal associations, or habitual timing structures can all strengthen situational activation because the nervous system learns predictive relevance relationally rather than abstractly.

A situational craving says as much about context as about the object itself.

Compensatory cravings become clearer once pressure states become visible. Fatigue, stress, emotional overload, glucose instability, sleep debt, appetite pressure, boredom, cognitive strain, frustration, or unresolved tension increase the motivational value of pathways associated with interruption, decompression, stimulation, familiarity, or rapid state change.

The craving intensifies because the system is attempting to offset strain.

This distinction matters because compensatory cravings are often interpreted morally rather than structurally. The nervous system under pressure naturally prioritizes what appears behaviorally regulating. The craving gains emotional force because the anticipated outcome seems capable of making the present condition easier to tolerate.

Relief-seeking is not the same as weakness.

Reinforced craving loops become easier to recognize through recurrence, predictability, familiar sequencing, and rapid activation. The nervous system begins retrieving the pathway efficiently because repetition lowers activation threshold. A relatively small cue can reactivate a much larger anticipatory structure involving reward expectation, memory, relief prediction, and response readiness.

The pathway feels automatic because it has been repeatedly practiced.

Recognition does not require suspicion or obsessive self-monitoring. This chapter is not proposing self-surveillance, behavioral policing, or endless analysis of every internal signal. The purpose is interpretive clarity, not control architecture.

Recognition changes the question.

Instead of asking, "What is wrong with me?" the nervous system can be interpreted through structural questions: What kind of signal pattern is active? Is this context-linked? Pressure-amplified? Intermittent? Reinforced through repetition? Organized around anticipated relief? Activated by fatigue or stress? Emerging from environmental availability?

Recognition reduces moral compression.

This distinction is critical because cravings become emotionally heavier when all signals are interpreted through a single framework of discipline, failure, weakness, or virtue. Different structures require different explanations even when they produce similar emotional intensity.

Interpretive clarity reduces unnecessary moralization.

Pattern recognition also improves stability because the nervous system becomes more readable. A situational craving no longer appears random once context activation becomes visible. A compensatory craving becomes more understandable once strain amplification becomes apparent. A reinforced loop becomes clearer once repetition and automaticity are recognized structurally rather than morally.

The signal becomes easier to interpret once its architecture becomes visible.

Importantly, recognition is not diagnosis. These categories are not fixed identities or clinical conditions. A person is not "a compensatory craver" or "a reinforced-loop person." The categories describe signal structures, not personalities. The purpose is descriptive organization rather than identity assignment.

Recognition clarifies the pattern without labeling the person.

This preserves the systems-based frame of the book. Cravings are not treated as moral verdicts or permanent traits. They are dynamic signals shaped by interacting pressures, contexts, learned associations, reinforcement histories, emotional states, metabolic conditions, and environmental structures.

The same person may experience entirely different craving patterns under different conditions.

A mild occasional craving during stable conditions may become compensatory under stress load. A situational pattern may become reinforced through repetition. Sleep debt may amplify emotional salience. Fatigue may increase the attractiveness of familiar low-friction reward pathways. Appetite pressure may intensify specificity. Memory may reactivate familiar relief architecture.

The nervous system continuously reorganizes around changing conditions.

Pattern recognition therefore improves interpretation because it separates structure from moral judgment. Cravings become less confusing when their organizing dynamics become visible. The signal no longer needs to collapse into one simplistic explanation involving weakness, lack of control, emotional failure, or "just hunger."

Different structures produce different kinds of urgency.

Seen clearly, craving stability begins with clearer interpretation rather than harsher judgment. Not every craving emerges from the same pathway. Some are occasional and transient. Some are situational and context-linked. Some are compensatory responses to pressure and strain. Some are reinforced loops strengthened through repetition and familiarity.

Recognition creates clarity without diagnosis.

A craving becomes more understandable when the nervous system's organizing pattern becomes visible. The signal stops appearing random, morally loaded, or personally indicting once occasional, situational, compensatory, and reinforced structures are separated conceptually. The craving remains real, but the interpretation becomes more precise, less confused, and less burdened by moral explanation.

Loop Weakening Mechanism

Reinforced craving loops often appear permanent while they are highly active because the pathway has become efficient, familiar, rapidly retrievable, and repeatedly reinforced across multiple systems simultaneously. The sequence begins to feel structurally fixed because activation occurs quickly, cue recognition becomes automatic, anticipated relief arrives early in the process, and the nervous system repeatedly rehearses the same predictive route toward reward, regulation, or interruption of discomfort.

But reinforcement intensity is not fixed.

Craving loops strengthen and weaken according to how often amplification systems continue converging around the same pathway. A highly active loop can feel psychologically inevitable while the nervous system is continuously refreshing the sequence through cue exposure, relief association, repetition density, emotional relevance, stress amplification, fatigue reactivity, and predictive salience. When those amplification conditions decrease, the loop often loses intensity gradually because the nervous system stops strengthening the pathway at the same rate.

This is the Loop Weakening Mechanism.

The Loop Weakening Mechanism describes the process by which reinforced craving pathways lose activation strength, automaticity, salience, and retrieval efficiency when amplification conditions decrease across cue exposure, reinforcement repetition, internal pressure, predictive relevance, and relief association. The pathway becomes less dominant because fewer systems continue assigning high importance to the same predictive sequence.

A loop weakens when fewer conditions continue strengthening it.

This distinction matters because craving reduction is often framed through moral struggle, behavioral victory, discipline, or force. But reinforced pathways do not weaken because a person "defeats" the craving. The nervous system simply stops receiving the same density of converging reinforcement signals across time.

The architecture changes because the reinforcement environment changes.

Strong craving loops often contain overlapping amplification systems operating simultaneously. Cue repetition repeatedly refreshes activation readiness. Memory restores familiar reward prediction. Emotional association increases salience. Stress amplifies relief value. Fatigue lowers tolerance for friction. Appetite pressure increases reward relevance. Glucose instability increases urgency. Sleep debt reduces emotional margin. Availability lowers response effort. Reinforcement repetition strengthens automaticity.

The loop gains strength because multiple pressures converge around the same pathway repeatedly.

This convergence explains why certain cravings feel unusually immediate or emotionally persuasive during periods of accumulated strain. The signal is not necessarily strong because one factor dominates. The signal becomes powerful because many amplification layers repeatedly reinforce one another at the same time.

Density matters more than isolated intensity.

When fewer amplification systems remain active simultaneously, the loop often begins losing force gradually. The nervous system stops assigning the same urgency, salience, or predictive importance to the pathway because fewer conditions continue refreshing its relevance.

Signals lose intensity when amplification layers stop converging.

Internal state stabilization is one of the most important weakening influences because craving intensity often depends heavily on unresolved pressure. When stress load decreases, sleep becomes more restorative, recovery strain softens, appetite pressure settles, energy availability stabilizes, emotional overload decreases, or fatigue becomes less dominant, the nervous system frequently assigns less urgency to pathways associated with rapid interruption, immediate relief, or fast state change.

The craving loses force because the surrounding pressure loses force.

This process does not require conscious suppression of desire. The nervous system simply stops treating the pathway as urgently necessary under conditions of lower amplification pressure. A reward sequence repeatedly associated with emergency regulation, decompression, stimulation, or rapid restoration often becomes less emotionally dominant when the surrounding system no longer carries the same intensity of unresolved strain.

Urgency decreases when pressure decreases.

Importantly, this chapter is not describing optimization tactics or self-improvement strategies. Internal stabilization is being described structurally rather than prescriptively. The nervous system under lower strain naturally evaluates reward salience differently than a nervous system operating under fatigue, overload, instability, or chronic stress amplification.

The pathway changes because system conditions change.

Cue exposure reduction also influences loop weakening because repeated environmental contact preserves activation readiness. A highly exposed pathway remains easy to retrieve because the nervous system continues encountering reminders, contextual associations, sensory exposures, routines, or environmental structures that repeatedly refresh predictive memory.

Repeated exposure keeps retrieval fast.

When cue density decreases, the pathway receives fewer opportunities for activation rehearsal. The nervous system stops refreshing the sequence at the same frequency. Familiarity may remain, but immediacy often decreases because the pathway no longer receives constant environmental reinforcement input.

Exposure frequency influences retrieval frequency.

A pathway repeatedly encountered remains psychologically near the surface. A pathway encountered less often gradually becomes less behaviorally immediate because the nervous system stops receiving repeated reminders to restore the sequence.

Availability preserves salience through repetition opportunity.

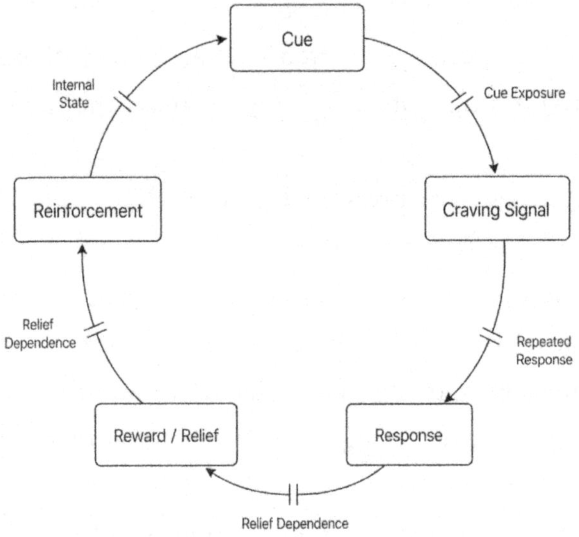

[Figure 18: Loop Weakening Points]

The weakening points illustrated in the figure matter because reinforced loops usually lose strength through multiple small reductions in amplification density rather than through dramatic elimination. Cue exposure may decrease. Reinforcement repetition may become less frequent. Relief association may weaken. Internal pressure may soften. Salience amplification may decline. Predictive relevance may narrow.

The loop weakens because fewer layers continue refreshing the same sequence repeatedly.

Repetition interruption contributes strongly to this process because automaticity depends heavily on rehearsal density. A pathway repeatedly activated becomes behaviorally efficient because the nervous system practices retrieval over and over again. The sequence becomes increasingly familiar, increasingly rapid, and increasingly easy to assemble.

Reinforcement requires repetition density.

When the sequence runs less frequently, retrieval efficiency gradually decreases because the nervous system stops strengthening the association at the same pace. The pathway may still exist clearly in memory, but activation speed, emotional immediacy, and predictive centrality often diminish over time as reinforcement density declines.

Familiarity can remain while urgency decreases.

This distinction matters because weakening is often misunderstood as erasure. Reinforced pathways do not necessarily disappear completely. The nervous system may continue recognizing the sequence long after the loop loses much of its prior dominance. Recognition and salience are not identical processes.

A remembered pathway is not always a highly active pathway.

Relief-seeking separation further contributes to weakening because many loops gain strength through repeated association between reward response and interruption of discomfort. Stress, overload, boredom, fatigue, emotional strain, appetite instability, cognitive pressure, sleep debt, and internal tension increase the perceived value of pathways associated with rapid decompression or tolerability.

The loop strengthens because the nervous system repeatedly learns, "this pathway changes the state."

When relief becomes less dependent on the same repeated reward route, the craving pathway often loses predictive centrality. The nervous system gradually stops assigning exclusive regulatory importance to that sequence because the same pathway no longer functions as the dominant or repeatedly rehearsed route toward interruption of discomfort.

Relief association weakens when regulation becomes less concentrated around one pathway.

This is not therapeutic reframing or behavioral coaching. The point is structural. Craving loops often remain highly active because the nervous system repeatedly treats the same sequence as behaviorally important for relief, stabilization, decompression, interruption, familiarity, or rapid state change. When that concentration decreases, predictive relevance frequently decreases alongside it.

The pathway loses urgency when it loses centrality.

Weakening is also usually gradual rather than dramatic. Reinforced loops rarely disappear suddenly because nervous systems preserve familiarity long after reinforcement density decreases. The pathway often remains recognizable while becoming less behaviorally dominant.

The signal becomes quieter before it becomes absent.

A person may still recognize the cue, remember the association, anticipate the sensory profile, or understand the prior reward pathway even while the craving loses urgency, emotional intensity, retrieval speed, or automatic activation strength.

Reduced activation probability matters more than total elimination.

This gradual shift often reflects reduced retrieval frequency. A pathway repeatedly retrieved remains highly available because the nervous system continuously refreshes the sequence. A pathway retrieved less frequently gradually becomes less immediate because retrieval rehearsal declines across time.

Retrieval efficiency weakens when rehearsal density weakens.

This does not require memory erasure. The nervous system may continue recognizing the pathway clearly while assigning it lower salience, less urgency, reduced emotional importance, or decreased predictive weight.

Memory can persist after dominance decreases.

Importantly, weakening often reflects broader stabilization across systems rather than direct suppression of craving itself. When stress softens, fatigue decreases, appetite pressure stabilizes, sleep improves, glucose urgency declines, cue exposure decreases, reinforcement frequency drops, and emotional overload becomes less central, fewer amplification layers continue converging around the same sequence.

The craving pathway loses force because the surrounding systems stop amplifying it simultaneously.

This explanation preserves structural neutrality. Loop weakening does not make a person morally superior, psychologically stronger, or more disciplined. The nervous system remains reward-responsive and predictive regardless of whether specific pathways strengthen or weaken.

Human reward systems do not disappear when specific loops lose intensity.

Some loops also remain highly persistent because reinforcement conditions remain continuously active. High cue exposure, repeated accessibility, chronic stress load, persistent fatigue, sleep debt, appetite instability, emotional overload, repeated relief reinforcement, low-friction reward availability, and repeated memory activation continuously refresh the pathway and preserve salience.

Persistence often reflects reinforcement density rather than personal defect.

This distinction prevents both moral judgment and unrealistic simplification. Reinforced loops are not permanent by definition, but neither are they instantly reversible through force or intention alone.

Their intensity reflects how frequently amplification systems continue refreshing the sequence across time.

The nervous system strengthens what it repeatedly rehearses.

Weakening therefore changes activation probability rather than eliminating reward responsiveness itself. The person remains capable of desire, pleasure prediction, sensory interest, anticipation, and reward-oriented behavior because those functions are part of ordinary nervous system organization.

The system remains predictive even when specific loops weaken.

Seen clearly, craving loops become more understandable when viewed as reinforcement systems rather than moral failures. A loop weakens when fewer layers repeatedly amplify the same predictive sequence. Reduced cue exposure, lower reinforcement density, decreased internal pressure, softened relief association, reduced salience amplification, and lower retrieval frequency gradually reduce activation strength across time.

The signal becomes quieter because the system stops strengthening it at the same intensity.

Automaticity decreases because repetition decreases. Salience declines because urgency declines. Retrieval slows because reinforcement density weakens. The pathway may remain recognizable while becoming less behaviorally central because fewer systems continue assigning high predictive importance to the sequence.

The loop weakens structurally rather than morally.

Understood this way, weakening reflects changing reinforcement conditions rather than victory, failure, purity, discipline, or transformation. The nervous system simply stops amplifying the same pathway with the same frequency, urgency, and convergence density. Over time, the sequence loses some of its immediacy because the surrounding systems stop repeatedly refreshing its dominance.

Stability Integration Mechanism

Craving stability is not the absence of desire. It is not permanent emotional neutrality around food, total removal of reward sensitivity, elimination of pleasure, or perfect insulation from wanting. Human nervous systems remain predictive, reward-responsive, sensory-oriented, emotionally associative, and metabolically adaptive across ordinary life. Desire continues to exist because reward signaling continues to exist.

Craving stability instead reflects a change in amplification.

A reward signal becomes less behaviorally dominant when fewer systems continue intensifying the same pathway simultaneously. The craving may still appear, but the signal often becomes less urgent, less repetitive, less emotionally concentrated, and less structurally amplified because the surrounding systems stop assigning such high converging importance to the same predictive sequence.

Stability does not erase desire. It reduces amplification.

This distinction matters because craving instability is often interpreted through moral language rather than systems language. Repetitive or emotionally intense cravings are commonly treated as evidence of weak discipline, defective restraint, addictive personality, emotional failure, or lack of control. But the intensity of craving often reflects convergence across multiple amplification systems rather than moral weakness within the person.

A signal becomes louder when more systems amplify it simultaneously.

This is the Stability Integration Mechanism.

The Stability Integration Mechanism describes the process by which craving pressure becomes less urgent, less repetitive, and less behaviorally dominant when reward signals, internal state, cue exposure, reinforcement density, recovery capacity, and environmental friction stop amplifying the same pathways at high intensity. Stability emerges not through suppression of reward systems, but through reduced convergence across amplification layers.

The opposite of craving instability is not control. It is lower convergence.

Craving emerges through interaction between reward prediction, appetite pressure, glucose regulation, fatigue state, stress load, sleep recovery, environmental exposure, reinforcement repetition, memory reactivation, relief expectation, and cue association. No single layer fully explains the signal. The craving becomes most intense when several systems repeatedly organize around the same anticipated pathway simultaneously.

The nervous system integrates pressures rather than isolating them.

This is why cravings can feel emotionally singular even when structurally multilayered. A person may experience one urgent craving while fatigue, stress, sleep debt, appetite instability, repeated cue exposure, reinforcement history, emotional strain, and anticipated relief are all contributing amplification simultaneously beneath the surface.

The signal feels unified because the amplification converges.

Reward signaling remains central to this process because the nervous system continuously predicts possible state changes associated with pleasure, relief, familiarity, stimulation, comfort, decompression, restoration, or emotional interruption. Cravings become especially persuasive when the predicted reward appears highly relevant to current conditions.

Prediction organizes motivational relevance before action occurs.

But reward signaling alone does not fully determine craving intensity. Appetite pressure strongly influences amplification because broad biological pressure increases the force assigned to reward-related pathways. Hunger, unstable satiety, delayed intake, perceived scarcity, or unresolved appetite tension can increase the motivational significance of reward-associated signals.

A craving gains force when appetite pressure supplies additional urgency.

This does not mean appetite pressure creates every craving. The nervous system can generate highly specific reward signals in the absence of substantial hunger. But when broad intake relevance combines with specific reward prediction, the signal often becomes more emotionally persuasive because general pressure and targeted anticipation begin reinforcing one another.

Broad pressure strengthens specific direction.

Glucose regulation contributes similarly because perceived instability in fuel availability increases the value of rapid state change. When energy feels unstable, the nervous system often assigns higher motivational importance to pathways associated with quick restoration, immediacy, sensory intensity, or fast perceived relief.

Instability changes the emotional value of speed.

Under conditions of stable fuel availability, a reward signal may remain interpretable and psychologically manageable. Under perceived glucose instability, the same pathway may acquire additional urgency because the nervous system increasingly prioritizes rapid restoration and reduction of uncomfortable instability.

Urgency rises when availability feels uncertain.

Stress load further amplifies craving salience because stress narrows tolerance and increases the perceived value of decompression, interruption, comfort, familiarity, or emotional softening. The nervous system under elevated strain becomes increasingly attentive to pathways associated with rapid regulation because unresolved pressure makes relief more behaviorally relevant.

Stress increases the emotional importance of immediate reward.

This does not mean stress creates all cravings, nor does it mean reward pathways are inherently pathological under strain. It means stress changes salience weighting. Relief becomes more valuable when pressure becomes more difficult to tolerate.

The craving intensifies because relief gains value.

Sleep debt and fatigue amplify the same dynamics through reduced capacity. Poor recovery narrows emotional margin, increases impulse pressure, lowers tolerance for friction, heightens reward sensitivity, and reduces reflective distance. Fatigue increases the attractiveness of low-effort pathways because cognitive, emotional, and behavioral effort all become more expensive under reduced recovery conditions.

A tired system values ease differently than a rested system.

This interaction matters because cravings often become more behaviorally persuasive under sleep debt or fatigue not because the reward itself fundamentally changed, but because the nervous system's ability to tolerate strain, delay, uncertainty, or effort changed substantially.

Capacity influences salience.

A craving stability framework therefore cannot isolate reward from recovery. Sleep, fatigue, stress, emotional strain, appetite regulation, and metabolic stability continuously shape how reward signals are interpreted and prioritized within the nervous system.

The signal never exists independently from system state.

Environment and repetition add another layer because availability, exposure frequency, response friction, and repeated reinforcement opportunities strongly influence activation density. A highly accessible pathway repeatedly encountered across ordinary environments receives more opportunities for cue activation, memory retrieval, anticipated relief, and reinforcement rehearsal.

Exposure frequency changes activation probability.

Repeated low-friction pathways become increasingly familiar because the nervous system repeatedly refreshes the same predictive architecture. The sequence becomes behaviorally efficient through repetition density. Cue recognition accelerates. Retrieval becomes faster. Anticipation arrives earlier. Familiarity increases emotional trust in the predicted outcome.

Repetition increases loop efficiency.

This helps explain why craving intensity often reflects interaction between internal state and environmental structure rather than either layer alone. A stressed, fatigued, poorly recovered nervous system repeatedly encountering highly accessible low-friction reward cues experiences more amplification opportunities than a rested nervous system under lower strain with reduced cue exposure density.

Systems converge contextually.

Memory and reinforcement deepen the same architecture because prior reward experiences preserve predictive associations across time. The nervous system remembers not only the object, but also the emotional tone, relief sequence, sensory profile, contextual setting, and anticipated state change associated with the pathway.

Memory restores relevance rapidly.

Reinforcement repetition strengthens retrieval efficiency because repeatedly rehearsed sequences become increasingly easy to reactivate. A familiar cue can retrieve an entire predictive structure involving reward expectation, emotional association, anticipated relief, sensory specificity, and response readiness.

The pathway gains speed through rehearsal density.

Craving stability therefore emerges partly through reduced amplification across these overlapping systems rather than through elimination of reward itself. Desire may remain present while urgency decreases. Pleasure may remain meaningful while repetition density declines. Reward sensitivity may continue while emotional dominance weakens.

Craving stability means the signal has less surrounding pressure.

This distinction between desire and urgency is central. Desire is a normal feature of predictive nervous systems. Desire may remain flexible, context-sensitive, intermittent, and behaviorally non-dominant. Urgency becomes more likely when multiple amplification layers converge around the same pathway repeatedly and intensely.

Desire can exist without high amplification.

A person may still enjoy sensory reward, anticipate pleasurable experiences, recognize familiar cues, or remember rewarding pathways without those signals becoming emotionally overwhelming, behaviorally dominant, or continuously urgent.

The nervous system remains reward-responsive even under stable conditions.

What changes under greater stability is the density of amplification surrounding the signal. Fewer systems continuously intensify the pathway simultaneously. Appetite pressure decreases. Stress salience softens. Sleep improves. Fatigue narrows less dramatically. Cue exposure loses density. Reinforcement frequency declines. Relief pathways diversify. Retrieval becomes less automatic. Salience becomes less concentrated.

The signal becomes easier to interpret because fewer layers are amplifying it simultaneously.

This does not create emotional neutrality or permanent absence of craving. Reward systems remain active because they are part of ordinary nervous system organization. The goal is not detachment from pleasure, absence of desire, or emotional purity around food.

Human reward systems do not disappear under stability.

Instead, craving stability reflects greater coordination across systems. Reward prediction becomes less amplified by simultaneous metabolic instability, emotional overload, fatigue reactivity, stress salience, sleep debt sensitivity, environmental repetition, and reinforcement density.

Stability emerges when amplification decreases.

This framework also preserves interpretive neutrality. Craving stability is not evidence of superior character, higher discipline, or moral success. Instability is not evidence of failure. The nervous system continuously reorganizes around changing pressures, capacities, environments, reinforcement histories, and recovery conditions.

The system changes as convergence changes.

A craving may feel highly dominant during periods of accumulated strain because multiple amplification layers become active simultaneously. The same pathway may feel substantially quieter under conditions of lower pressure, improved recovery, reduced reinforcement density, and lower cue saturation because fewer systems continue strengthening the sequence at once.

Intensity reflects convergence more than virtue.

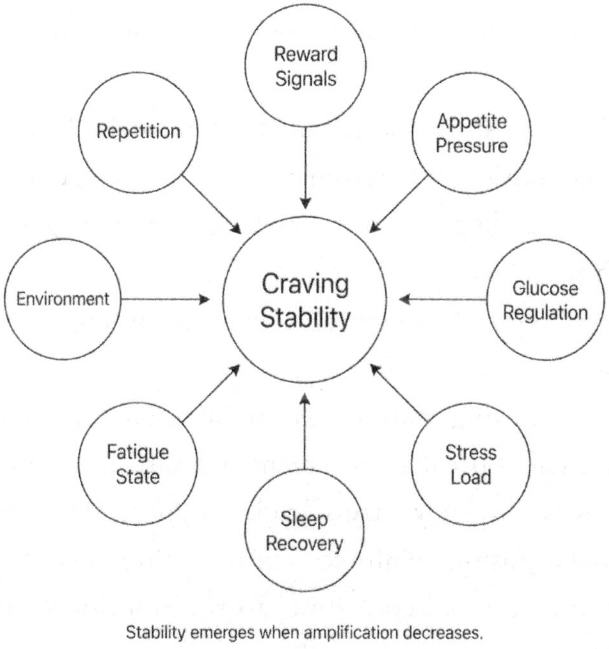

[Figure 19: Craving Stability Integration Model]

The integration model matters because it shows craving stability as coordination across interacting systems rather than conquest over desire. Reward signals remain present. Appetite continues functioning. Memory persists. Environmental exposure still exists. The nervous system remains predictive and responsive. But amplification decreases when fewer systems repeatedly intensify the same pathway simultaneously.

The signal becomes less dominant because the system stops assigning such concentrated importance to it.

This also explains why craving stability often feels less emotionally dramatic than instability. Highly amplified systems produce urgency, repetition, emotional concentration, attentional narrowing, and rapid retrieval. Lower amplification produces greater interpretive distance because fewer layers continuously push the signal toward behavioral centrality.

Reduced convergence creates more psychological space around the signal.

The craving may still appear, but it often carries less urgency, less emotional compression, less automaticity, and less repetitive activation because the surrounding systems are no longer amplifying the pathway at the same density.

The pathway remains recognizable while becoming less behaviorally central.

Seen clearly, craving stability is an integrated systems outcome rather than a self-control achievement. Reward prediction, appetite pressure, glucose urgency, stress load, fatigue state, sleep recovery, environmental exposure, reinforcement repetition, memory activation, and relief expectation all contribute to the emotional intensity and behavioral dominance of craving pathways.

Craving stability emerges when those amplification systems stop converging around the same sequences at high intensity.

Desire remains possible.

Pleasure remains possible.

Reward remains meaningful.

But the signal becomes less urgent, less repetitive, less behaviorally dominant, and easier to interpret when fewer layers continuously reinforce the same predictive pathway. The nervous system remains reward-responsive while operating under lower amplification density, lower convergence pressure, reduced reinforcement intensity, and greater overall coordination across systems.

Craving Stability as System Coordination

Craving stability is not the disappearance of desire. It is not the removal of appetite, reward sensitivity, pleasure, sensory interest, memory, or wanting. Human nervous systems remain predictive, associative, reward-responsive, and context-sensitive across ordinary life. Signals continue to arise because prediction continues to operate. Reward remains meaningful because reward systems remain part of normal regulation, learning, adaptation, and behavior.

Craving instability begins when amplification intensifies around specific pathways.

A reward signal becomes increasingly dominant when multiple pressures repeatedly converge around the same anticipated response. Appetite pressure, glucose urgency, stress load, fatigue, sleep debt, emotional strain, cue exposure, environmental accessibility, memory reactivation, reinforcement repetition, and relief expectation can all organize around the same predictive sequence simultaneously. The signal gains urgency because the surrounding systems continue assigning importance to the same pathway.

Craving stability therefore reflects reduced amplification rather than elimination of reward.

This distinction matters because cravings are often interpreted morally rather than structurally. Intense cravings are frequently treated as evidence of weak discipline, defective restraint, emotional failure, addictive personality, or lack of character. But craving intensity is often better understood as the output of converging pressures within a predictive nervous system than as evidence of personal weakness.

The signal becomes louder when more systems amplify it at once.

Cravings do not emerge from a single layer. They are shaped through interaction between reward prediction, sensory memory, anticipated relief, cue association, appetite state, fatigue, stress salience, sleep quality, fuel stability, repetition density, environmental exposure, and reinforcement history. The nervous system continuously evaluates conditions in relation to expected outcomes, available relief pathways, and predicted state changes.

A craving becomes especially persuasive when the system predicts that a specific response may rapidly alter the current state.

That alteration may involve pleasure, decompression, familiarity, stimulation, emotional interruption, comfort, reduced strain, perceived restoration, or relief from instability. The pathway gains force because the nervous system increasingly treats the anticipated response as behaviorally relevant under current conditions.

Prediction organizes urgency before action occurs.

This is why cravings often feel emotionally immediate even before any response takes place. Anticipated reward becomes psychologically active before the outcome itself exists. The nervous system begins organizing around expected relief, expected comfort, expected restoration, or expected decompression before the response occurs physically.

The craving is often about the predicted state change as much as the object itself.

Cue-driven repetition intensifies the same architecture because repeated exposure preserves activation opportunities. Familiar environments, routines, emotional states, screens, social settings, times of day, sensory patterns, and transition points repeatedly reactivate predictive pathways associated with reward or relief. The pathway gains familiarity because it continues being rehearsed.

Repetition increases retrieval efficiency.

A cue repeatedly paired with reward does not merely remind the nervous system of the response. It helps restore the predictive structure surrounding the response. Memory retrieves emotional tone, sensory association, anticipated relief, contextual familiarity, and expected reward simultaneously. A small cue may reactivate an entire sequence because the pathway has become behaviorally efficient through repetition density.

Familiarity increases activation speed.

This efficiency is not evidence of moral failure. It reflects reinforcement architecture. A sequence repeatedly rehearsed becomes easier to retrieve because the nervous system learns through repeated association. Cue, craving, response, reward, relief, and reinforcement become increasingly linked through repetition across time.

The system remembers pathways that repeatedly appear relevant.

Compensatory reward seeking deepens the same process because cravings often intensify when reward pathways become associated with reduction of discomfort. Stress, fatigue, sleep debt, boredom, emotional strain, overload, appetite pressure, glucose instability, restlessness, or internal tension increase the value of rapid state change. The nervous system under pressure becomes more attentive to pathways associated with interruption, decompression, familiarity, or relief.

Relief can reinforce a pathway as strongly as pleasure.

This does not make relief-seeking pathological. Nervous systems naturally move toward reduction of strain and away from unresolved pressure. The important distinction is structural rather than moral. A pathway becomes increasingly dominant when the nervous system repeatedly learns that a specific response appears capable of rapidly softening discomfort or changing state.

The loop gains force because relief gains relevance.

Fatigue and sleep debt intensify this process because reduced recovery narrows tolerance, increases reward sensitivity, lowers emotional margin, and raises the value of low-friction pathways. Stress amplifies salience because pressure increases the importance of rapid decompression. Appetite instability amplifies reward because unresolved intake pressure increases motivational intensity. Glucose urgency sharpens immediacy because unstable fuel availability increases the perceived value of rapid restoration.

Multiple systems can amplify the same pathway simultaneously.

When convergence becomes dense, cravings often feel emotionally compressed, behaviorally urgent, repetitive, and difficult to interpret clearly. The signal begins to dominate attention not necessarily because the reward itself changed, but because surrounding systems continuously strengthen its salience.

Urgency reflects amplification density.

Desire and urgency are not the same process.

Desire may remain flexible, contextual, intermittent, and interpretable. Human beings continue wanting pleasurable experiences under stable conditions because reward sensitivity remains part of ordinary nervous system organization. Craving instability emerges when desire becomes narrowed by urgency, reinforced repetition, compensatory pressure, and repeated cue activation.

Desire can exist without behavioral dominance.

This distinction is central to craving stability because the goal is not emotional neutrality around reward. The nervous system does not stop being predictive or reward-responsive under stable conditions. Pleasure remains meaningful. Appetite remains functional. Sensory preference remains human. Memory remains active.

Craving stability does not require desire to disappear.

What changes under greater stability is the amount of surrounding amplification attached to the signal. Fewer pressures repeatedly intensify the same pathway simultaneously. Stress salience softens. Appetite pressure decreases. Recovery improves. Fatigue reactivity lowers. Reinforcement density declines. Cue exposure becomes less dominant. Relief pathways become less concentrated around the same repeated responses.

The signal becomes quieter because fewer systems continue strengthening it.

Craving stability therefore reflects coordination across systems rather than control over reward. The nervous system remains reward-responsive while operating under lower amplification density. Signals become more interpretable because they carry less convergence pressure around them.

A signal becomes easier to read when it is no longer amplified by every surrounding pressure.

This also changes the emotional meaning often assigned to cravings themselves. When cravings are interpreted exclusively through morality, intensity becomes confused with character. Strong signals appear to mean weak discipline. Repetition appears to mean failure. Relief-seeking appears to mean emotional defect. But structural interpretation changes the frame entirely.

The craving becomes understandable rather than condemnable.

A repetitive pathway may reflect reinforcement density, environmental exposure, memory retrieval, stress salience, fatigue reactivity, appetite instability, glucose urgency, sleep debt sensitivity, or repeated relief association rather than defective character. The nervous system is continuously adapting around prediction, repetition, pressure, and expected outcomes.

The signal reflects coordination across systems rather than simple personal virtue.

Craving stability emerges when amplification decreases across those systems simultaneously. Reward signals remain present, but they become less emotionally compressed, less repetitive, less urgent, and less behaviorally dominant because fewer pressures continuously intensify the same predictive sequence.

The opposite of craving instability is not control. It is reduced convergence.

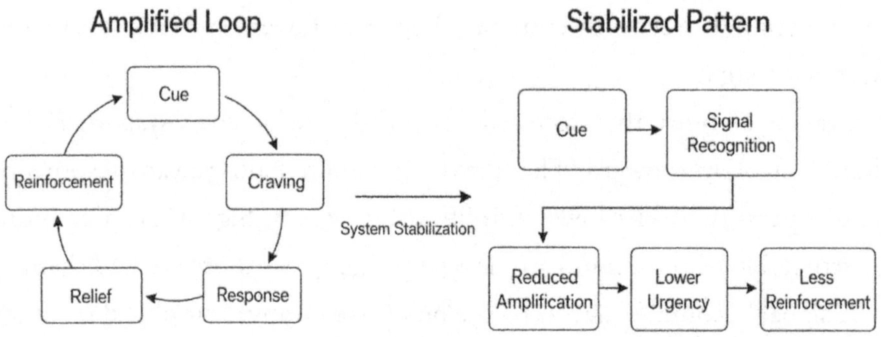

[Figure 20: Reinforced Signal Loop to Stability Model]

The transition from amplified looping toward greater stability is therefore not a transformation into a desireless state. It is a reduction in reinforcement density, urgency concentration, compensatory pressure, and repeated activation frequency. Familiar pathways may remain recognizable while losing some salience, automaticity, emotional intensity, or retrieval speed because the nervous system stops amplifying them at the same level.

A loop weakens when fewer systems continue strengthening it.

This weakening is often gradual rather than dramatic. Reinforced pathways usually lose dominance through reduced amplification across time rather than through sudden elimination. The nervous system may still recognize the cue, remember the reward, or anticipate the experience while assigning it less urgency, less predictive centrality, and less behavioral importance.

Recognition remains possible even when dominance decreases.

Craving stability therefore does not require suppression of reward systems, erasure of memory, removal of pleasure, or permanent absence of desire. Stability reflects lower convergence across reinforcement systems. Reward remains part of human regulation, but the signal becomes less compressed by urgency, less burdened by repeated amplification, and less morally loaded in interpretation.

The goal is not control over craving. The frame is coordination around the systems that shape it.

Seen clearly, cravings become less confusing when interpreted as reinforced predictive signals shaped by pressure, context, repetition, recovery capacity, emotional state, and system coordination rather than as evidence of personal failure. The nervous system remains associative, reward-responsive, and adaptive throughout ordinary life. But when fewer amplification layers repeatedly converge around the same pathways, the signal often becomes quieter, more interpretable, less urgent, and less behaviorally dominant across time.

Craving stability emerges not from elimination of desire, but from reduced amplification surrounding it.

About the Author

Nathan Reed writes about metabolic stability in systems exposed to load, variability, and time.

His work examines how biological capacity is shaped by energy availability, recovery architecture, sleep amplitude, muscle mass, environmental demand and workload. Rather than treating nutrition, fasting, sleep, and training as isolated tactics, he approaches them as interacting regulatory systems governed by margin, buffering, oscillatory coherence, and constraint dominance.

The Stability framework explores how physiological compression accumulates gradually and how proportional calibration preserves long-horizon resilience across decades. The objective is not peak optimization, but preservation of functional continuity under load.

Craving Stability is part of a broader metabolic stability ecosystem developed under Perennial Publishing, each volume addressing a distinct vector of biological durability.

The work is designed for readers who prefer structural clarity over motivational rhetoric and long-horizon coherence over short-term intensity.

The Metabolic Stability Series

Metabolic Stability – (Cornerstone Volume)
Fasting Fundamentals – (Foundational Volume)
Intermittent Fasting
Prolonged Fasting
Electrolytes
Insulin Stability
Glucose Stability
Metabolic Flexibility
Appetite Stability
Energy Stability
Blood Sugar Stability
Fat Loss Stability
Fatigue Stability

Craving Stability

Additional Titles Include:

The Vitality Series:
Sleep and Recovery
Strength and Aging
Hormones & Sexual Health

Part of a Broader Stability Framework

The Metabolic Stability Series is part of a larger stability ecosystem published by Perennial Publishing.

Related domains include:

Money Stability — structural durability in financial systems

Career Stability — positioning, load tolerance, and transition resilience

Mental Stability — cognitive steadiness under pressure and uncertainty

Emotional Stability — regulatory steadiness in environments that do not slow down

Foundations — low-fragility life architecture

Vitality — energy, strength, and biological function across time

Each domain approaches stability as a structural problem: capacity versus load, buffering versus shock, governance versus drift. Together, they form a unified framework for long-horizon durability across the major systems that shape human trajectory.

About Perennial Publishing

Perennial Publishing produces practical systems guides for building stability in an unstable world.

Our books explore the foundations of long-term resilience across health, finance, career, and everyday decision-making. Each title focuses on clear frameworks, durable principles, and practical strategies that help readers build lasting stability rather than short-term fixes.

The Perennial catalog includes series on metabolic health, financial stability, career systems, and personal consistency. While each book stands on its own, they share a common goal: helping individuals create durable systems that support a stable and sustainable life.

Made in the USA
Monee, IL
06 November 2026

68118397R00114